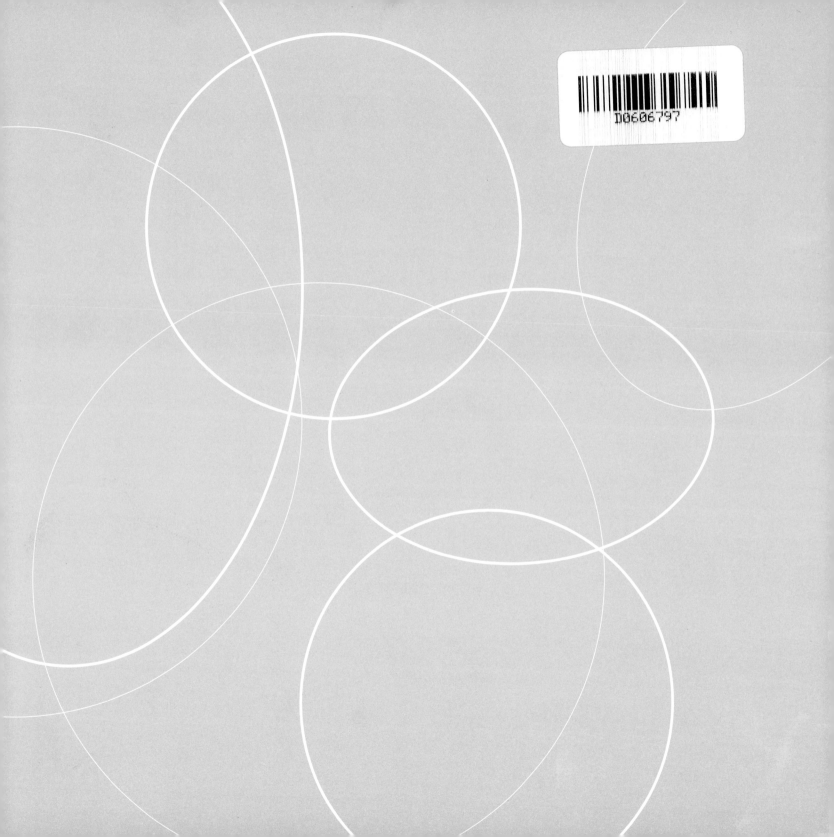

Sara Slavin | Karl Petzke

the art
of the bath

photography | Karl Petzke

art direction/styling | Sara Slavin

text | Stefanie Marlis

design | Morla Design

edible recipes | Sandra Cook

bath recipes | Gaylen Blankenship

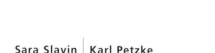

CHRONICLE BOOKS

SAN FRANCISCO

Library of Congress Cataloging-in-Publication Data
available. ISBN 0-8118-1645-1

Printed in United States of America.

Design and typesetting by Morla Design, Inc.,
San Francisco

Distributed in Canada by Raincoast Books
9050 Shaughnessy Street
Vancouver, British Columbia V6P 6E5

10 9 8 7 6 5 4 3

Chronicle Books LLC
85 Second Street
San Francisco, California 94105

www.chroniclebooks.com

Credits

"Haiku by Bashō" translated by Robert Hass in
The Essential Haiku by Robert Haas.
Reprinted with the permission of The Ecco Press.
Copyright ©1984 by Robert Haas.

Excerpt from *Zen Mind, Beginner's Mind*
by Shunryu Suzuki.
Reprinted with permission of Weatherhill.
Protected by copyright under terms of the International
Copyright Union.

"Gloire De Dijon" by D.H. Lawrence from
D.H. Lawrence Selected Poems.
Reprinted with permission of Viking Press.
Copyright © 1957 by Frieda Lawrence Ravegli.

"Each Bird Walking" by Tess Gallagher from
Amplitude: New and Selected Poems.
Reprinted with permission of Graywolf Press.
Copyright © 1987 by Tess Gallagher.

"Archaic Torso of Apollo" by Rainer Maria Rilke translated
by Stephen Mitchell in *The Selected Poetry of Rainer
Maria Rilke*.
Reprinted with permission of Random House, Inc.
Copyright © 1982 by Stephen Mitchell.

Nilus deMatran Architectural Design
(Bathroom on page 40)

Arnelle Kase for Barbara Scavullo Design
(Bathroom on page 59)

Douglas Burnham for Interim Office of Architects (IOOA)
(Bathrooms on pages 66 and 96)

Bibliography

1. *Pleasures of the Japanese Bath*, Peter Grilli,
Weatherhill, New York, 1992.

2. *Sauna, The Finnish Bath*, H. J. ViherJuuri,
The Stephen Green Press, Brattleboro, Vermont, 1965.

3. *An Irreverent and Almost Complete Social History of
The Bathroom*, Frank Muir,
Stein and Day, New York, 1982.

4. *The Medical History of Waters and Spas*,
Roy Porter, ed., Wellcome Institute For The
History of Medicine, 1990.

5. *Baths and Bathing in Classical Antiquity*,
Fikret Yegül, The Architectural History Foundation
and The MIT Press, New York, 1992.

6. *Rodale's Illustrated Encyclopedia of Herbs and Plants*,
Rodale Press, Emmaus, Pennsylvania, 1987.

7. *How to Take a Japanese Bath*, Leonard Koren, Stone
Bridge Press, Berkeley, California, 1992.

8. *Undesigning the Bath*, Leonard Koren, Stone Bridge
Press, Berkeley, California, 1996.

Acknowledgements

The elements needed for a perfect bath are simple: water and you. But the elements needed to create a book are much more complex and numerous.

The following people and places have been indispensable to us in making this book happen, and we thank them.

We got tremendous support and encouragement from Nion McEvoy, Christina Wilson, Michael Carabetta, and Pamela Geismar at Chronicle Books.

Jennifer Morla and the staff at the office of Morla Design continue to design books that are always inventive, surprising, elegant, and visionary.

Creating a text both poetic and informative was accomplished with great ability and generosity by writer Stefanie Marlis.

The challenge of creating recipes that are both soothing and refreshing for the bather was left in the most capable hands of Sandra Cook, who met the challenge in a most delicious and imaginative way.

The task of gathering herbs and flowers from the garden and spice cabinet and turning these ingredients into magical bath potions was met by Gaylen Blankenship who has given this book potions both practical and sensuous.

So many of the beautiful things in this book were graciously loaned to us by some of the Bay Area's most wonderful businesses and we thank them so much for their ongoing generosity: Summerhouse, Mill Valley, CA; David Luke and Associate, S.F.; Sue Fisher King, S.F.; Waterworks, S.F.; Dandelion, S.F.; and especially Iris Fuller, Robert Perez, and Michael Potter from Fillamento, S.F.

We also offer our gratitude and thanks to the following for providing us with our fabulous locations: James Allen at the Public Affairs office of Hearst Castle; A. Peter Sallick of Waterworks; Peter VanDine Architecture & Light; Arnelle Kase of Barbara Scavullo Design; Jim Jennings Architecture; Kabuki Hot Springs, S.F.; Interim Office of Architects (IOOA); Post Ranch Inn, Big Sur; and Nilus deMatran Architectural Design. We wish to thank the generosity and support of the following homeowners: Leslie Becker, Joan Boyd, Mitzi Johnson, Zachery Smith, Jennifer Morla and Nilus deMatran, Chiquita Woodard, Kathleen and Peter VanDine, and Gaylen and Ed Blankenship.

Our thanks go, as well, to Anne Culbertson and the staff of Morla Design, Hennessey Knoop for her great contribution and assistance to Stefanie Marlis, Allyson Levy for her assistance to Sandra Cook, and Wendi Nordeck for her assistance in the studio and on location.

We would also like to say thank you to the following for support, information, inspiration, and generosity: Leonard Koren, Vic Zauderer, Ed Galvez, and Jeff Long.

With love always to Mark Steisel, Sybil Slavin, Kate Slavin, and Lillian Moss.   ~ S.S.

All my love to Mari and Alanna.   ~ K.P.

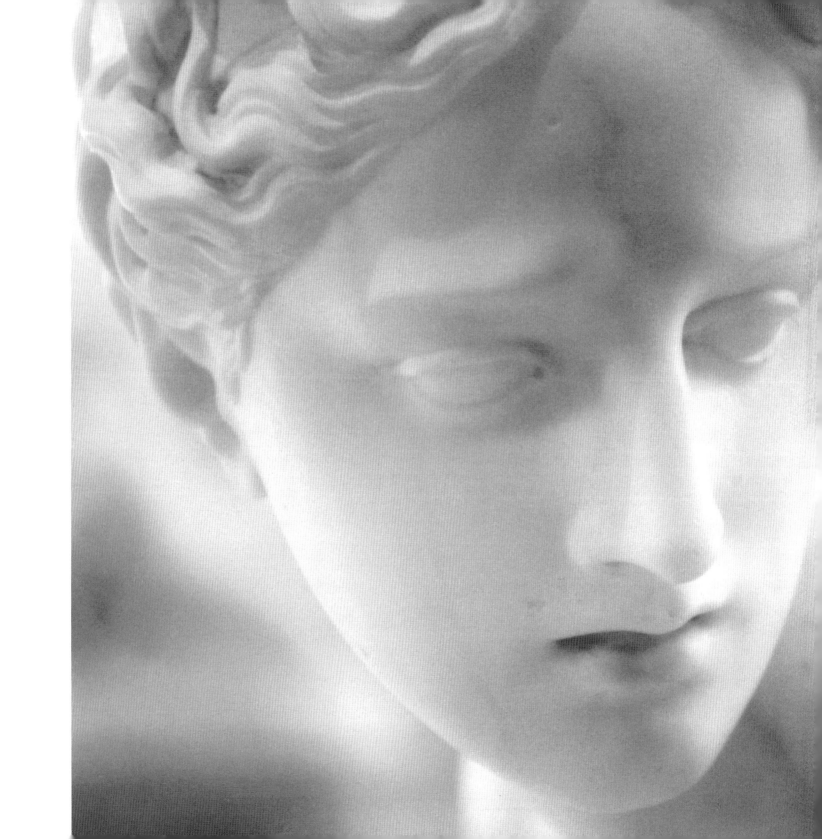

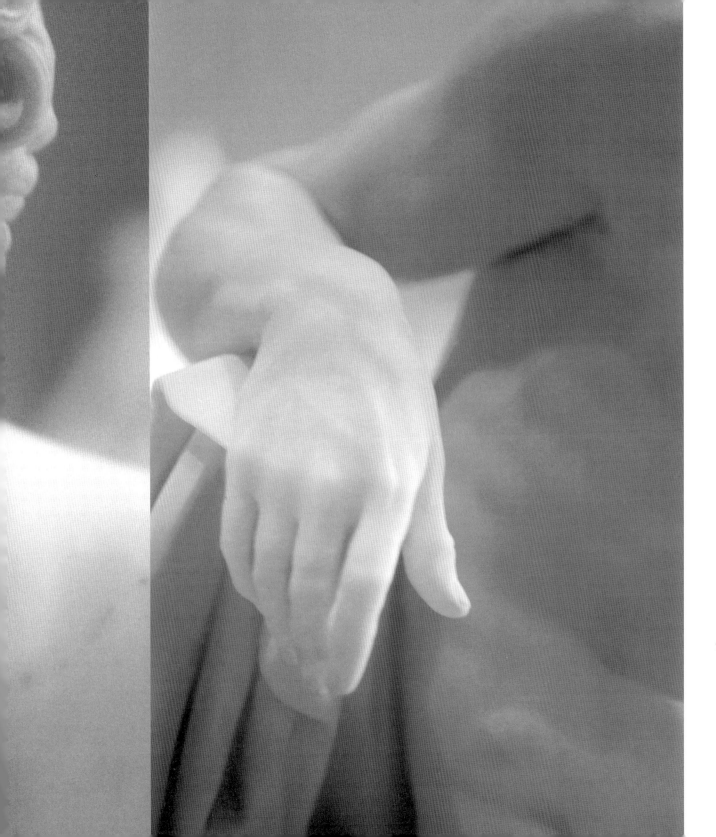

senses

"Coming home, don't bathe,"

 said Napoleon to his wife, Josephine.

>   After months away, a man might well long to breathe in his

>   wife's pure scent. And living in an era when one bathed

>   only out of true necessity, the general no doubt knew what

>   a bath washed away but not what it gave back.

>   Lost on him was the higher purpose of bathing—

>   a profound sense of renewal,

>   which today, given the bristle and weight

>   of daily life, places the ritual

>   under the category of heaven on earth. The body and its muscles let go;

>   the mind wanders through open meadows;

>   and the spirit,

>   soothed by watery nothingness, rises.

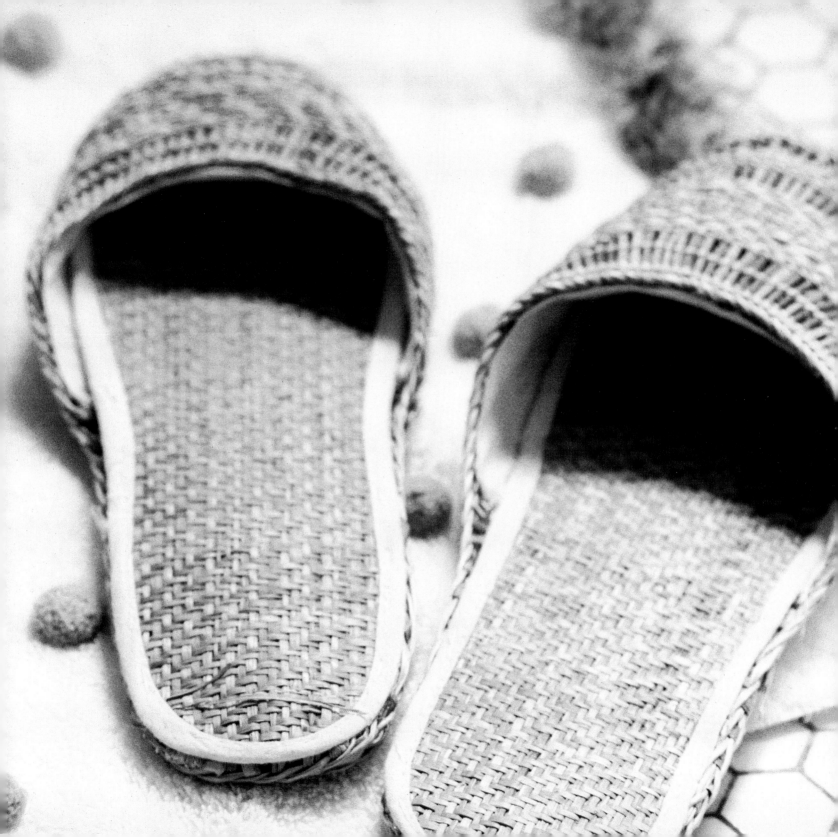

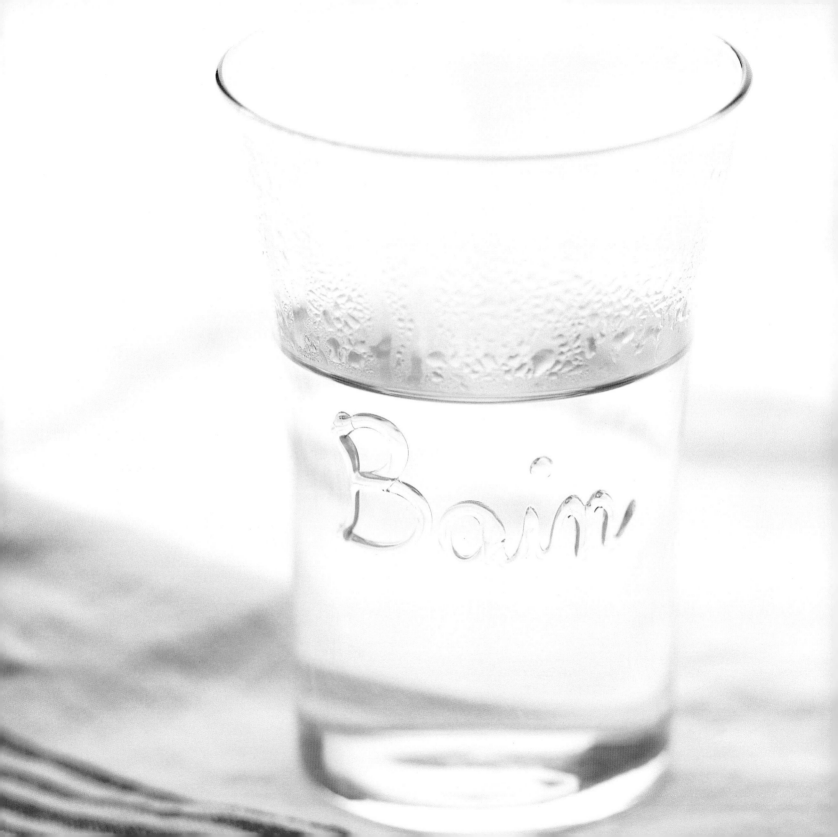

With a turn of the wrist, you open the tap, and it gushes forth, coming up through the pipes, humming with elemental vitality; it's a sound you'd know anywhere, rushing into the tub—merely itself, purely itself.

Letting it splash a little—on the back of your hand, on the floor. Testing it. Too warm? Too cold? Sailing the seas of the South Pacific, the ancient Polynesians navigated by the temperature of the currents. Gingerly, you extend a toe. You dip your hand, like a ladle, into this odorless, colorless elixir. Every original culture speaks of its transformative powers. Lap, lapping against the porcelain as you ease yourself into it, as you shift your weight. Or is it laughing? Pull the plug, clockwise, counterclockwise—a dimple running away to the other side of the world.

The steam rises, now fragrant and soothing; this clarity into which you have added a handful of salts and lavender and sage now reflects the sky through the open windows and the aquamarine of the 1930s tiles. "The seat of the soul," said Novalis, "is where the inner world and the outer world meet. Where they overlap, it is in every point of the overlap." You press a cool glass of it against your temple—water.

a history of bathing

Water—ambiguous, amorphous. In so many creation stories, water symbolizes a nothingness from which the gods bring forth the tangible. At once bright and pure, it is also a dark force, carving canyons, flooding plains, and swelling into shipwrecking waves. But whether positive or negative, water is the most basic element of life and therefore divine.

When the ancient Greeks wanted to be closer to the spirit, they bathed. In the earliest Greek mythology, the ancestral Earth gave birth to Heaven and to Pontos, the realm of the saltwater sea. Earth then coupled with Heaven, conceiving Okeanos, the father of all springs and rivers. Thus, the idea of heaven remained imminent within all waters.

In ancient Greek cosmology, waters constituted the limits of the universe—Earth lay like an island in the middle of their great expanse. It's notable that the Greeks attributed to water the enigmatic aspects of wisdom and knowledge. For it was the water gods who gave birth to daughters possessing qualities of intelligence—among them Metis, "prudence," Idyia, "the knowing one," and Panopeia, "the all-seeing one." Water with all its power had a very special place in the minds of the ancient Greeks, and so did bathing.

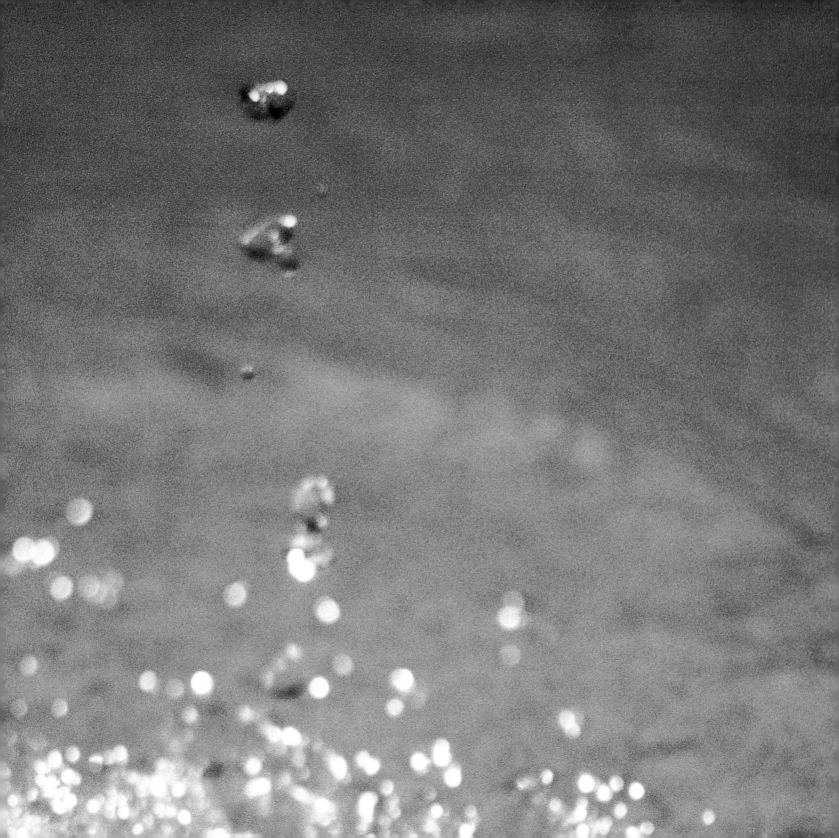

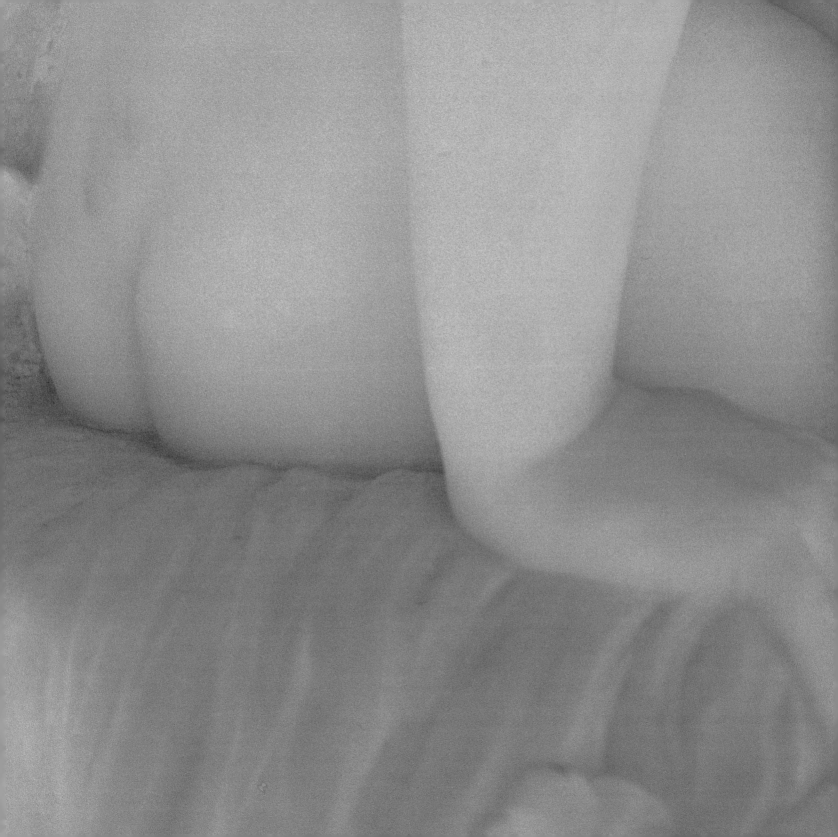

In Homer's age, bathing was believed to be healthy and rejuvenating—elevated to such an extent that it was considered a special reward for heroes, warriors, gods, and kings. We see this in *The Odyssey* when Circe bathes Odysseus upon his arrival to her island: "When the bright copper [cauldron] was boiling, she sat me down in a bath and washed me with water from the cauldron mixed with cold to a comfortable heat, sluicing my head and shoulders till all the painful weariness was gone from my limbs. My bath done, she rubbed me in olive oil, and clothed me in a fine tunic."

The first known bathtub was found in Crete in the great palace at Knossos, most likely built for the legendary King Minos around 1700 B.C. The Minoans invented impressive technologies that provided water for this tub, including a system of interlocking terra-cotta pipes.

Ancient medicine determined that physical exercise and bathing were not only a means to good health but ways to bridge mind and body. Washing and bathing facilities were integrated in the Greek *gymnasium*, a place where one went to compete, socialize, debate, philosophize, and relax. In the earliest *gymnasia*, athletes performed cold water ablutions in the *loutron*—an open-air space with fountains and basins. In later *gymnasia*, a pool was incorporated into the *palaestra*—a colonnaded enclosure for exercise—and decorative spouts were placed high up so the bather could shower. By the fourth century B.C., Greeks enjoyed bathing with hot water so much that many felt it had become a decadent activity.

While the Greeks initiated the rites of social bathing, the Romans perfected them. To be Roman was to bathe. Much like today's health club, baths were popular venues for socializing. The *thermae*, which were truly grand, state-built bathhouses, had libraries, lecture halls, cult shrines, porticos, and promenades as well as a *palaestra* and tracks for exercise and games. In the fourth century A.D., Rome had many hundreds of small public baths, eleven magnificent *thermae*, more than 1,350 public fountains and cisterns, as well as hundreds of private baths. The average Roman used three hundred gallons of water a day—nearly what an American family of four uses today.

Though there were many baths that were exclusive, the majority of the more than 800 small baths and the eleven *thermae* were open to anyone who paid the small entrance fee; some baths charged nothing at all.

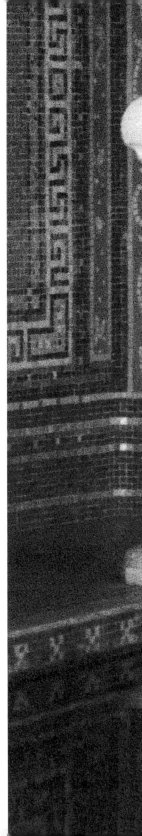

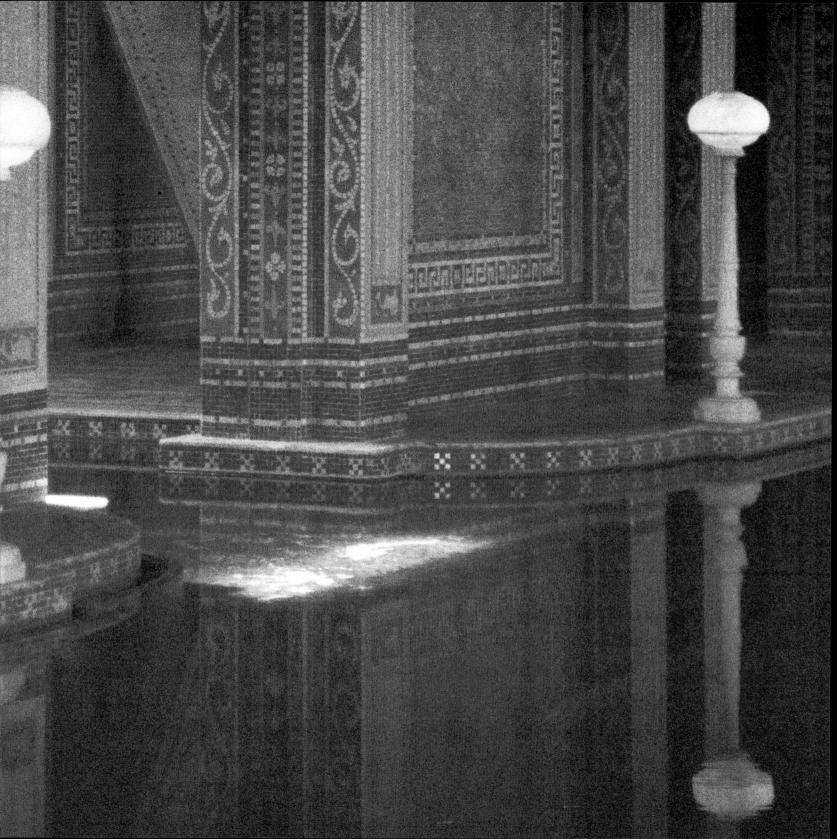

It was not unusual for a Roman Emperor to visit these public baths, enjoying a few hours among his people. As an institution, the baths created the illusion of a classless society where nearly everyone could enjoy one of the perks of the imperial system.

The Romans made bathing more luxurious than any other culture at any other time. High vaulted ceilings were decorated with rich marble veneers; there were silver basins and spigots, and bronze fountainheads. It's no wonder that the highlight of the Roman day was a visit to the baths. A wealthy Roman went to the public bath with his slaves, who carried his bathing paraphernalia: exercise and bathing garments, sandals, linen towels, and a toilet kit containing anointing oils and perfume in flasks, a *strigil* (a metal blade with a slightly curved end used to scrape down excess oil from the body), and, no doubt, a sponge. One Roman meeting another at the baths would offer a wish for good bathing, *"Bene lava!"* The baths were divided into chambers arranged by temperature: the *tepidarium*, a warm room, the *caldarium*, an even warmer room, the *aconicum*, the warmest of the three, and the *frigidarium*, a cold pool. Often, Romans began their dinners in the baths with a light snack and an aperitif.

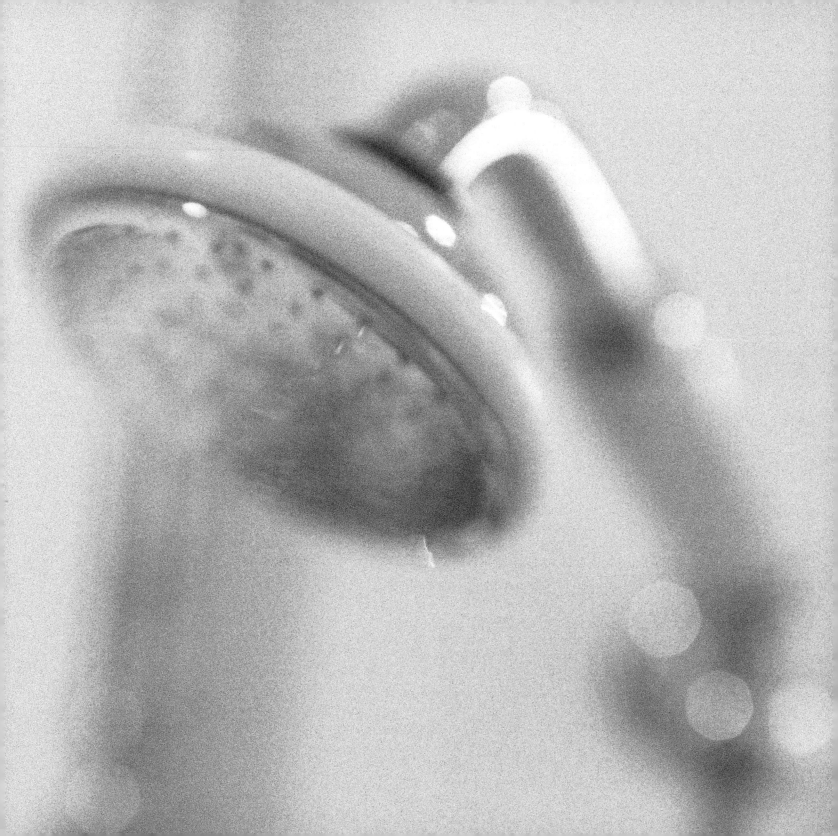

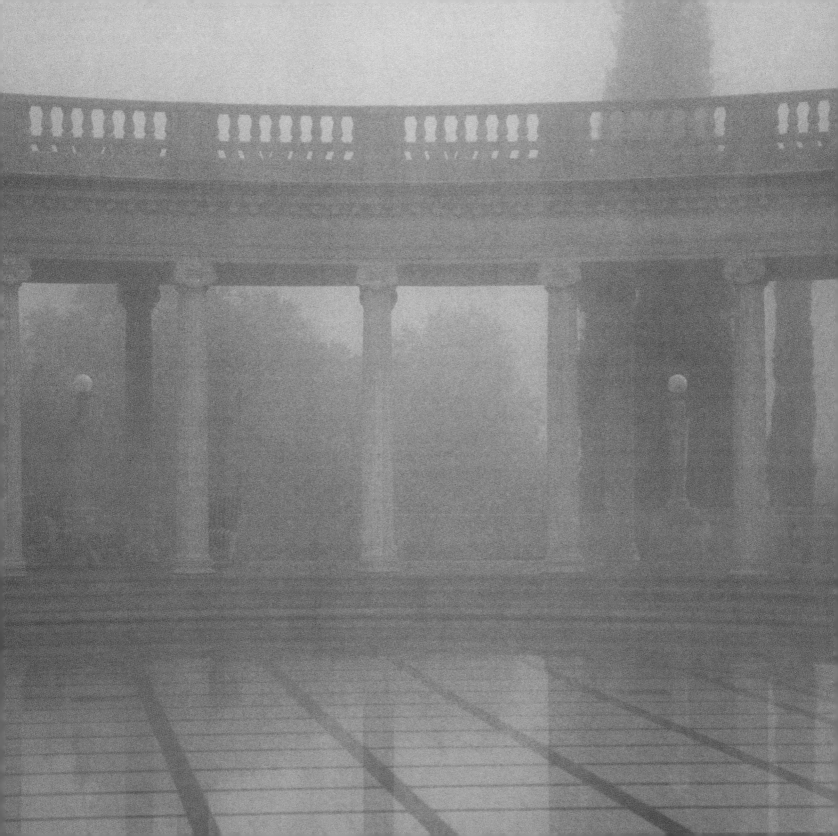

For a long time, women and men bathed separately. In Pompeii, men and women had completely separate facilities. But in the Roman baths, the sexes did eventually more than mix. Many of the most infamous baths were adjuncts to brothels. One might say the baths did anything but keep the Roman Empire clean, morally speaking. Emperor and philosopher Marcus Aurelius spoke of the baths with great disdain: "What is bathing when you think of it—oil, sweat, filth, greasy water, everything revolting...." The respected first-century thinker Seneca also condemned the baths, saying that they distracted young men, pulling them away from their military duties. For centuries, as the Empire waned, Christian critics also pointed to the sexual decadence and moral delinquency of the baths.

We cannot know his legendary head
with eyes like ripening fruit.
        And yet his torso is still suffused with brilliance from inside,
like a lamp, in which his gaze, now turned to low, gleams in all its power.
        Otherwise the curved breast could not dazzle you so, nor could
a smile run through the placid hips and thighs
        to that dark center where procreation flared.

Rainer Maria Rilke

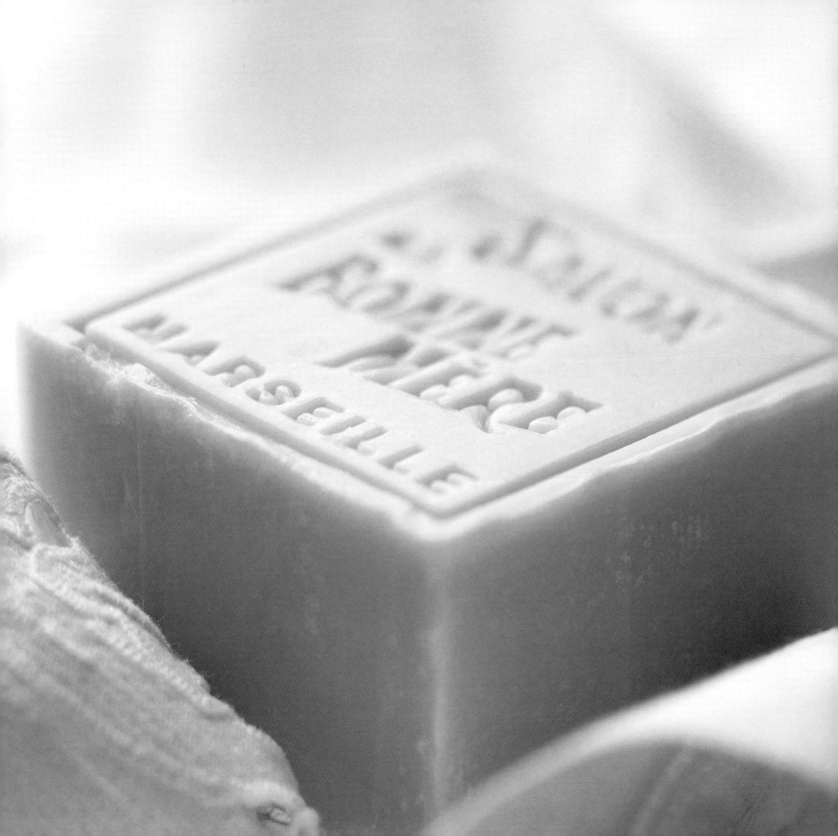

Until this century, Christians viewed cleansing the body and purifying the spirit as opposing acts. The Church, associating baths with the decadence of the Romans, disavowed bathing, and so discouraged the faithful from habits of cleanliness. "To those that are well, and especially to the young, bathing shall seldom be permitted," Saint Benedict ordered in the sixth century. Saint Francis of Assisi spoke of the unwashed body as a "stinking badge of piety." With the bathing practices of Greece and Rome cast aside, Europe went, as it's been said, "nearly a thousand years without a bath."

This attitude against cleansing the body is clearly reflected in the evolution of baptismal rites. Though John the Baptist submerged Jesus in the waters of the river Jordan, by the fourteenth century, baptism had become a symbolic act where purification was accomplished simply by the priest dousing a child or convert with a few drops of water. Immersing the body to wash away sin was no longer deemed necessary. However, while the Church discouraged the masses from baths and bathing, Christian monasteries, ironically, preserved ancient bathing practices. One monastery, Christchurch at Canterbury, had plumbing by the middle of the twelfth century; and the monks bathed in tubs of hot water several times a year.

For everyone else, how much or little one washed depended on one's class. The wealthy cleaned their hands, faces, and hair with a water jug and a shallow basin. But even so, Queen Isabella of Castille bragged that she had bathed twice in her entire life—once at birth and once before her wedding. Influenced by Turkish baths, the crusaders briefly reintroduced Europe to the technologies of public baths; however, these baths, which were most popular in France and England, were short-lived, as the Church was quick to determine that they promoted licentious behavior.

This ecclesiastical condemnation continued until the nineteenth century on both sides of the Atlantic. Colonial Americans were discouraged from bathing, as bathing inevitably led to nudity, and nudity most surely to promiscuity. For a time, residents in Philadelphia who bathed more than once a month risked being jailed. It was not until Science undermined the Church's absolute power that Western culture embraced bathing. So, whereas other cultures historically promoted cleansing the body as a way to bring the individual closer to the cosmos, Christians began bathing in the modern age because Science deemed it medically sound.

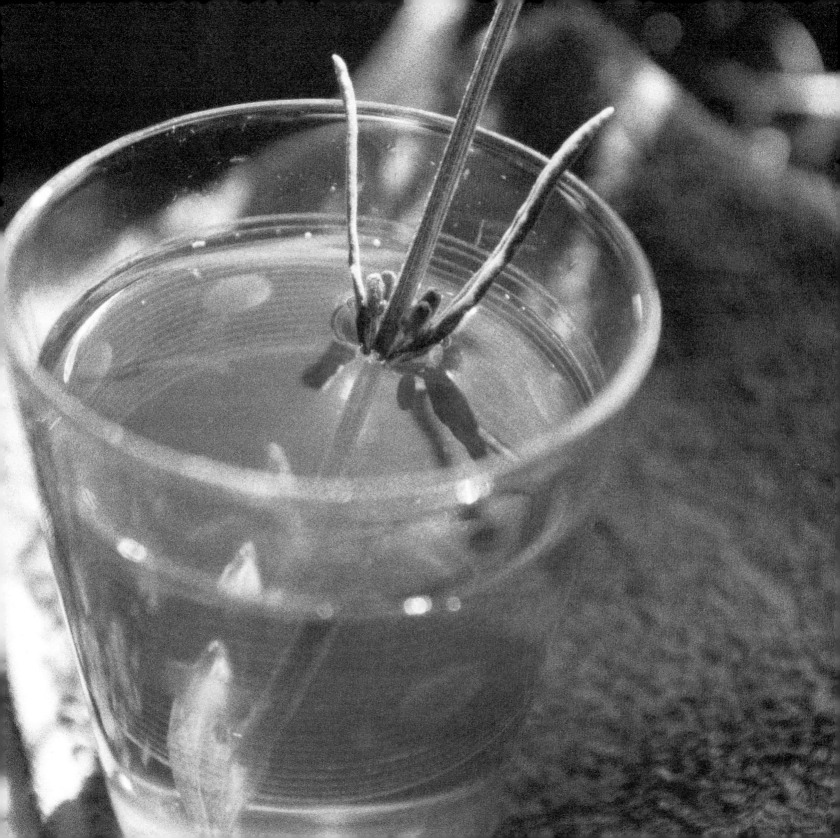

So it was that John Wesley, who believed cold water bathing cured more than fifty afflictions, from breast tumors to blindness, could sermonize that "cleanliness was next to Godliness." By 1853, similar thinking led the British Parliament to pass the Public Baths and Wash-House Act—it had become clear that unsanitary conditions led to disease. Apparently, the lords and ladies realized they were losing their workforce to a lack of cleanliness, and by 1860 London had more than ten public washhouses.

Meanwhile, in fashionable American households, portable tubs and the Saturday night bath were becoming popular. By World War I, reliable water heaters and built-in tubs and sinks put regular bathing within everyone's reach. Still, it took the "Cleanliness Crusade," launched by the Cleanliness Institute and linked to Proctor & Gamble, to really convince Americans that bathing daily was the right thing to do. Today, the average American bathes more than seven times a week.

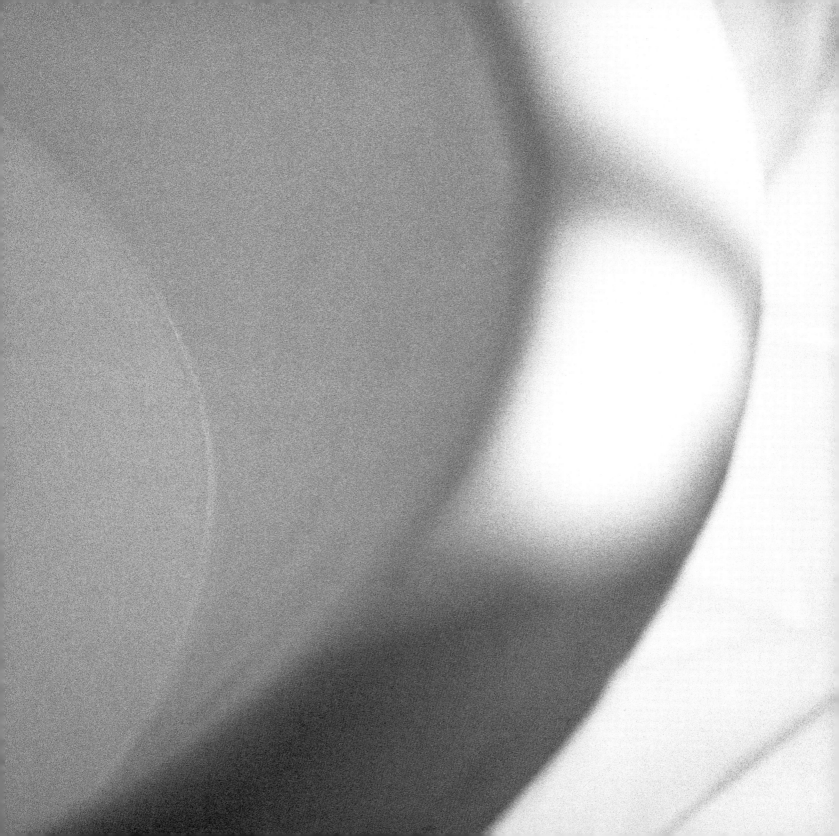

paraphernalia

On a visceral level bathing may be about letting go and letting the bath induce a feeling of deep relaxation. Physically, however, there are hundreds of ways that one can remove dirt, scrub away old skin, perfume, dry and generally pamper the body. It seems everyone has a favorite bathtime routine. One can soak in soaps, gels, oils, or salts. One can use an enzyme formula or a homemade scrub, a sponge, a loofah, nylon gloves, a washcloth, a brush, or a pumice stone. One can dawdle, toweling oneself in plush terry cloth, and then slip into a silk kimono, or follow one bath with another and air dry in the sun.

Every culture has had its own methods of renewal. Before exercising, the ancient Greeks and Romans anointed their naked bodies with olive oil and dusted themselves with sand. Afterward, they rubbed the sand off, removing outer layers of dead skin with it, and then, using a *strigil*, a metal blade with a slightly curved end, scraped off the excess oil before finally rinsing with fresh water. In the Roman toilet kit, a metal box called a *cista*, bathers packed anointing oils and perfumes, *strigils*, and sponges.

Waves enfolding
    a crescent of humble sand.
The river's seeming meandering
    as it carves away
canyons, alluvials, plains.

Rain on a slate roof,
    soft-spoken until tedious.

A still pool:
    a single fallen leaf in a
concentric spell.

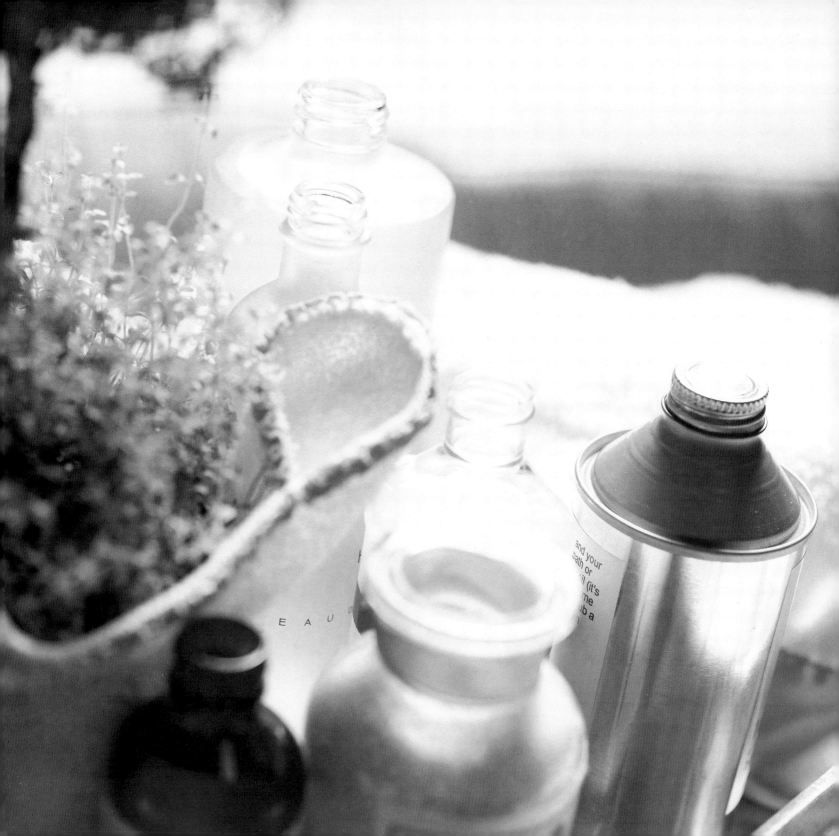

E A U

and your
bath or
il (it's
me
b a

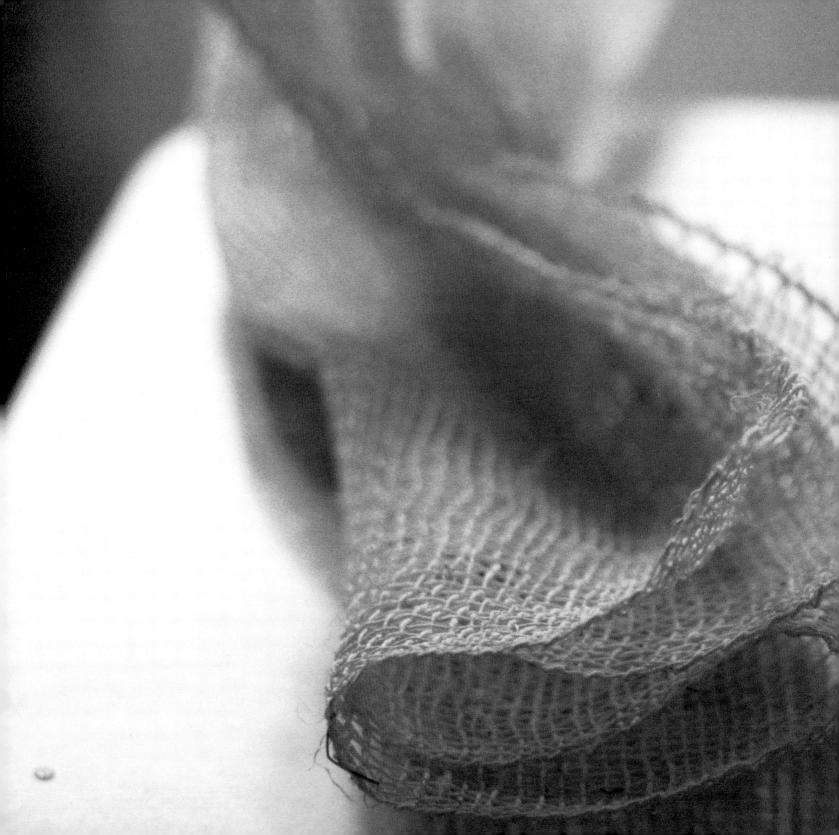

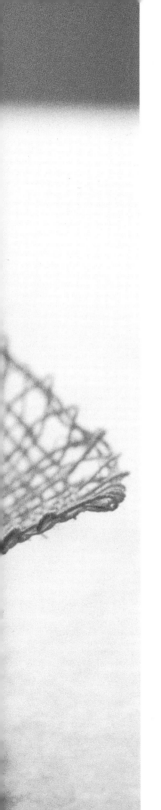

During the Ottoman Empire, the Turks went to the *hammam* or public bath, where the community gathered to cleanse, relax, and gossip in a sunlit steamroom. Using a long bristled brush, they whisked a rich olive oil soap and a little water together in a hammered copper bowl until the soap became a froth of creamy lather. With a softer brush, they combed the lather over their bodies. Finally, they scrubbed off the dead skin and impurities with a scratchy goathair mitt. To remove dead skin and hair from their bodies, Turkish women used *halawa*, a depilatory made with cooked sugar, honey, olive oil, and lemon, which softened the skin exquisitely. On the eve of her marriage every inch of a bride's body would be gone over with *halawa*.

And just as Turkish women made *halawa* from ordinary ingredients in their kitchens, you'll find that many of the foods in yours also contain enzymes for making natural, nonabrasive exfoliants: Papayas, with the enzyme papain, as well as apples, grapefruit, and pineapple all smooth and soften the skin. You can also make simple scrubs with anything from oatmeal to quinoa that will gently take away the top layers of dead skin.

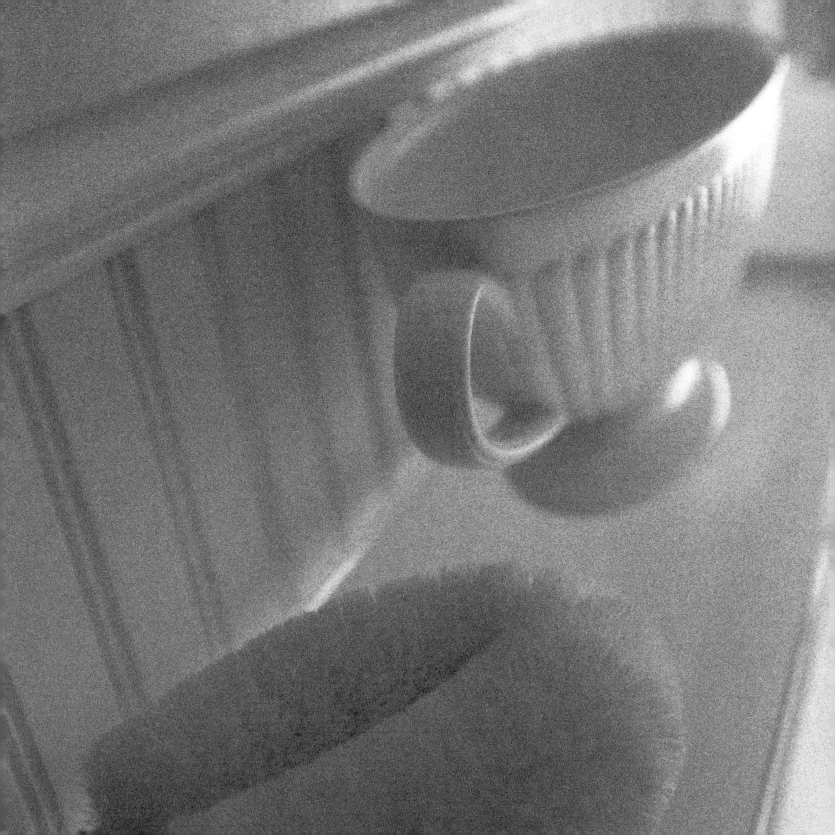

Sponges and loofahs are also wonderful exfoliators and have been used for centuries. Until the 1700s, people thought that sponges were solidified sea foam—an idea that may well have stemmed from the myth that Aphrodite, goddess of love and beauty, was created out of sea foam. Now we know that a sponge is the fossilized skeleton of a invertebrate sea animal.

Likewise, a loofah, which is a little rougher than a sponge, is made from the fibrous internal skeleton of a dried gourd, a plant related to the cucumber. A loofah, like a sponge, becomes softer when it gets wet. The open structure of the fibers allows air to pass through, so a loofah is less apt to grow bacteria than a sponge. When using either a loofah or sponge, it's best to massage the skin in a circular motion.

A pair of nylon gloves, found in bath specialty shops, is a nonorganic, but very efficient exfoliator. The effect is somewhere between a loofah and a washcloth. And gloves offer great flexibility, letting you easily massage every contour of your body.

Invented in 1900 by Cannon, the washcloth is ideal for more sensitive skin. A washcloth made from Egyptian cotton with its extra-long fibers is both soft and durable. It may be used, for instance, to exfoliate the upper arms, reducing the roughness caused by clogged pores. Another type of bath cloth is made from the fibers of the ayate cactus. Its wide, open weave makes the ayate cloth a superb exfoliator.

Natural bristle brushes are also excellent exfoliators, especially the long-handled kind that let you get at hard-to-reach places such as your back. Dry brushing before a bath is exceptionally invigorating. Begin at the ankles, always brushing toward the heart. The increased circulation lends a healthy glow to your skin. Brushes are frequently made with synthetics, but the softest and best are those made of natural boar bristles.

A relative of granite, pumice is a volcanic lava that solidified while it was still filled with gas bubbles—this accounts for its porous structure and light weight. Use a pumice stone to polish the calluses on your feet and hands. Be careful not to scrub too hard, however. Just scrub a little every so often, and after a time, you'll see real results. Many bath stores also offer a terra-cotta scrubber that emulates the effect of the natural pumice stone.

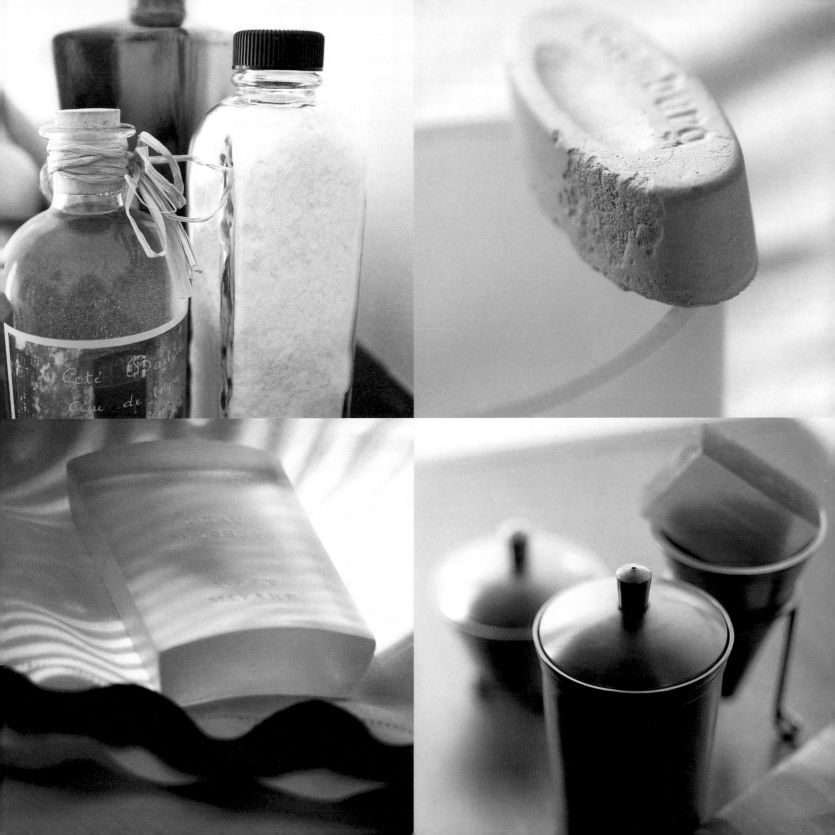

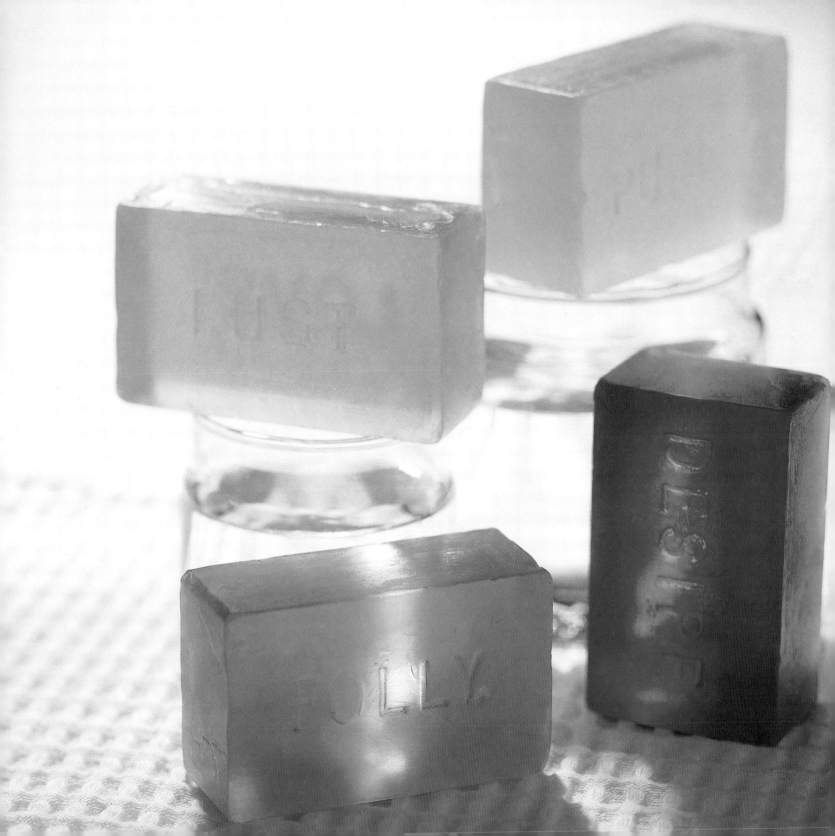

Soap's been on the scene since around 600 B.C., when the Phoenicians boiled fat or tallow in water, stirring in wood ash until the mixture hardened. The soap molecule has a cleaning action because it attracts oil and dirt while repelling water, causing dirt to loosen its bonds with the skin. Certainly, a rich, creamy lather does testify to having actively pursued an elevated state of cleanliness. The best soaps contain very little air and are milled in long cylinders, which are then hand-cut into bars. Soaps that are triple-milled—a French method—are both unusually dense and long lasting. These days many people prefer pure vegetable soaps to those made with synthetics or animal products.

However, others find that using soap daily causes their skin to feel dry and itchy. So if you're tired of the "bar" scene, you might try a "soapless" soap or a "gel." Soapless cleansing bars were invented during World War II, when shortages of natural ingredients forced chemists to invent synthetics. But today's trend is more au natural, with more and more gels being made with moisturizing botanicals such as jojoba and camellia oil as well as Vitamins A and E. Another solution to the dry skin conundrum is to only lather up certain places, such as underarms and feet.

Many beauty gurus warn against bathing too frequently because the skin doesn't have time to replenish its natural oils between baths. By adding botanical oils to the water, you can have your bath and smooth, healthy skin, too. Nut oils such as almond and avocado may be combined with scented herbal oils such as rose, lavender, or jasmine. It's best to soak a few minutes first, and then add the oil. Your skin will have had a chance to absorb moisture, and the oil will coat the skin, keeping the moisture in.

If you want your bath to be more like a retreat to a warm tropical sea, you might try adding the sea's own accessory—salt. Bath salts are used to soothe both irritated skin and aching muscles. The salts, to which seaweed extracts are often added, dilate pores, allowing the skin to absorb trace minerals and soluble vitamins. Many beauty stores carry products containing salts from the Dead Sea.

Later, showering,
my body—my parents' body—
gleaming.

Over the whole world likenesses:
offspring, yes, and die-cut widgets,
bing cherries, chocolates.

And everywhere one's family life,
one's solitude, one of a thousand thousand lakes.

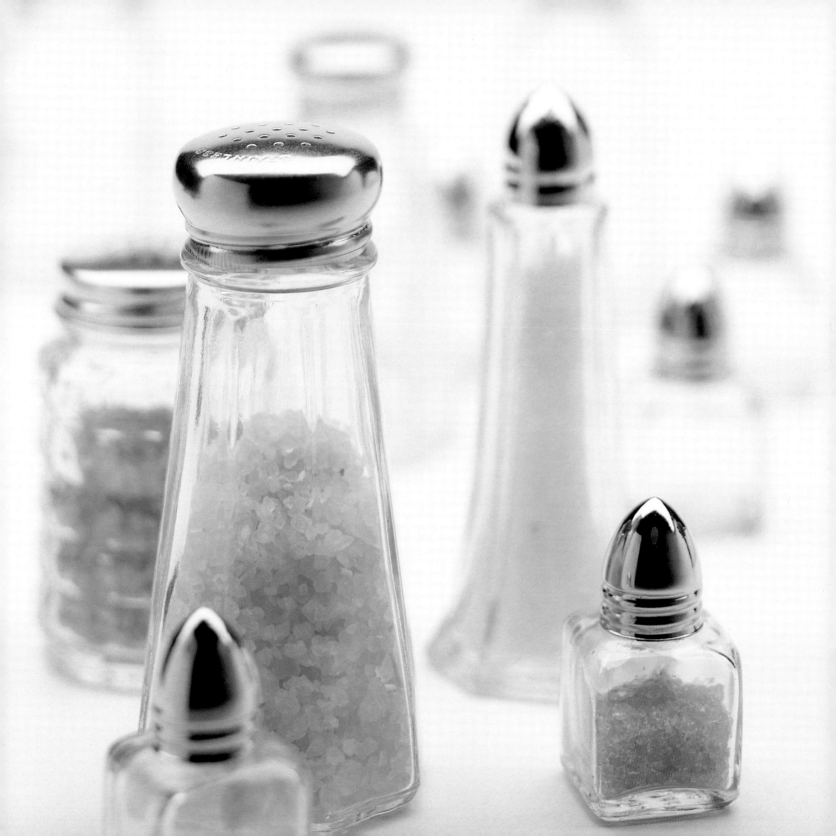

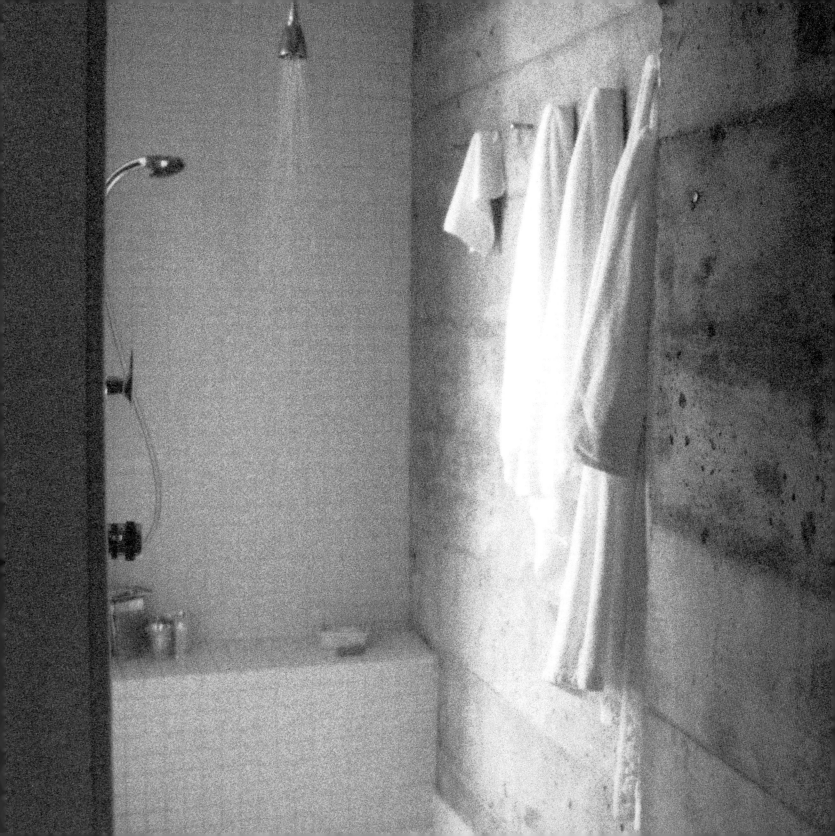

Fundamentally, a towel is just something to dry oneself with, but it can also be a grand finale to the bath. It helps if it's the kind of towel made from lustrous Egyptian cotton, longer than Isadora Duncan's scarf, hefty and infinitely absorbent—like the one J. Peterman wanted to steal the first time he stayed in that five-star hotel in Lugano. And white—whiter than the detergent you use to keep it white. Although…something can be said for walking away from the tub wrapped in shell pink or moss green.

From tub to towel to robe. White terry cloth is the classic, but no matter the color or fabric, a robe should offer refuge—almost like a bearish hug. It's a place to go when you're not quite ready for clothes. The silk kimono, the European waffle-weave robe, the traditional jacquard-woven robe, the à la-Hollywood chenille robe—all are equally suitable for après bath comfort.

an abbreviated glossary of fibers & weaves

Chenille In French, chenille means caterpillar; chenille is woven from a special yarn and has a thick, distinctive pile.

Combed Cotton Only the best grades of cotton are combed, a process that separates, straightens, and arranges the long, desirable fibers. The yarn spun from combed cotton is clean, smooth, and durable.

Dobby A special attachment for a loom, a dobby allows small geometric figures to be woven into a larger piece of fabric. On towels, the term refers to the decorative band that interrupts the terry weave.

Egyptian Cotton Grown in the Nile Valley since the time of the Pharaohs, this cotton is considered the premium variety because of its extra-long fibers, which produce a softer, more absorbent, and most durable fabric.

Jacquard Created on a Jacquard loom, this woven fabric is distinguished by an intricate, often classic pattern.

Pima Cotton Developed in Pima County, Arizona, this is a long-staple hybrid of American cotton crossed with Egyptian cotton. The finest Pima cotton is called Supima.

Terry Cloth Also known as "terry toweling" or "Turkish toweling," this fabric can be woven of cotton or a cotton-polyester blend. The deep pile on one or both of its sides makes it exceptionally absorbent.

Upland Cotton The most widely cultivated cotton in America, this variety of cotton has medium-length staples, producing a cloth that's soft, though of medium fineness.

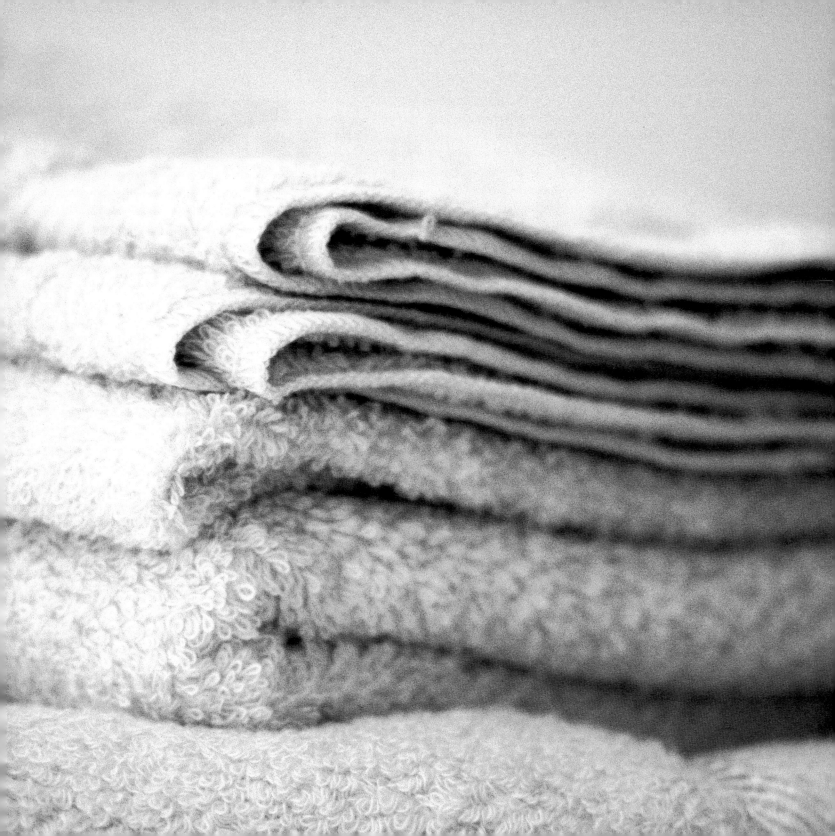

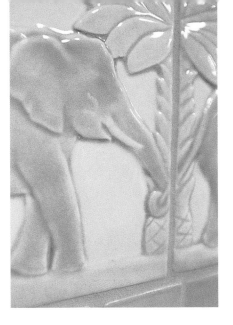

mango–passion fruit agua fresca with jicama ice

This is a smooth, topical, balmy, and easy-to-linger-with concoction. When the juice is gone, the jicama makes a fragrant and hydrating snack.

2 ripe mangos, peeled and seeded

1 passion fruit

¾ cup water

1 jicama, peeled

Roughly chop the mango. Cut the passion fruit in half and scoop out the soft pulp inside. Place the fruit and water in a blender and puree until frothy. Pour over frozen jicama cubes. Serves 2.

To make jicama ice cubes, cut the jicama into one-inch squares. Freeze for at least 20 minutes. This will make about 8 to 12 cubes, depending on the size of the jicama.

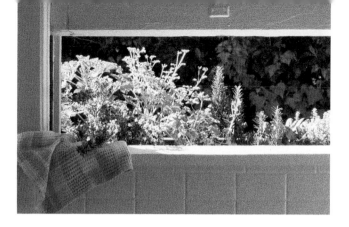

bath windowsill garden

Those in the city or the country lucky
enough to have a window in the bathroom
can grow a window sill garden containing
small amounts of herbs and flowers for the
bath. Just reach out the window and gather
a bouquet for your bath.

All-geranium: strawberry, orange, peppermint, rose, and lemon-scented geraniums.

Citrus mix: orange mint, lemon verbena,
calendula, miniature lavender.

Sweet herbal: pineapple mint, red sage,
lemon balm, and rosemary.

Floral: scented geranium, baby roses,
lavender, and calendula.

faucet wreaths

These little miniature wreaths, herbal or floral, will hang on the tub faucet. While you
are bathing, break off bits of these wreaths
and toss into tub.

Gather sprigs of favorite herbal or floral
bath enhancers, such as lavender,
chamomile, rosemary, or Cecil Brunner roses.
String chosen herbs and aromatic flowers on
thread or thin elastic and form into a small
circle, about five to seven inches. Circle
around tub faucet, or float in tub.

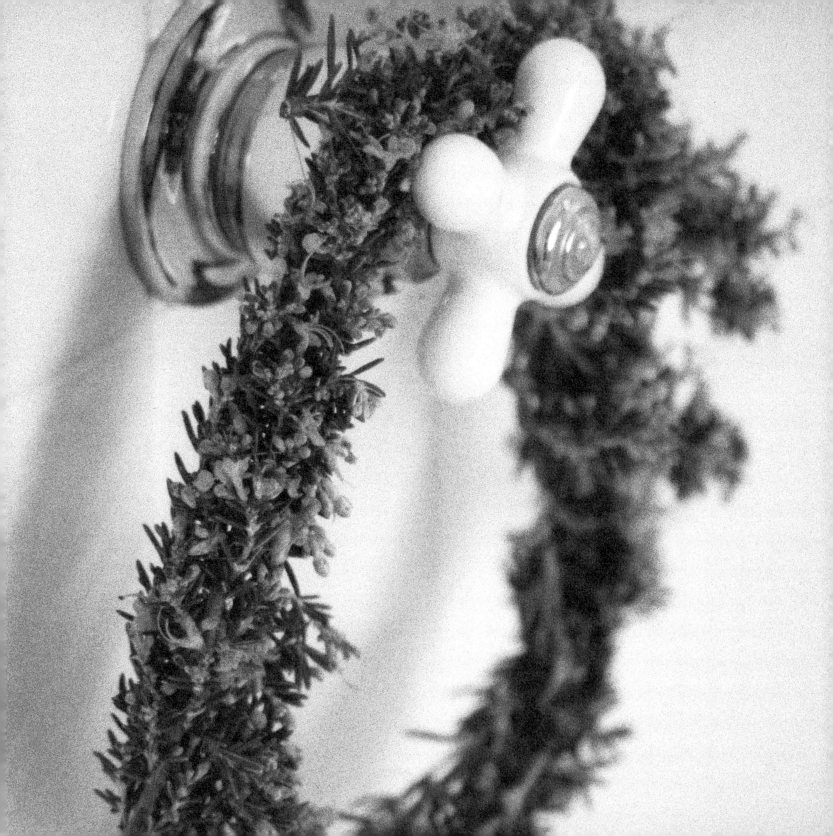

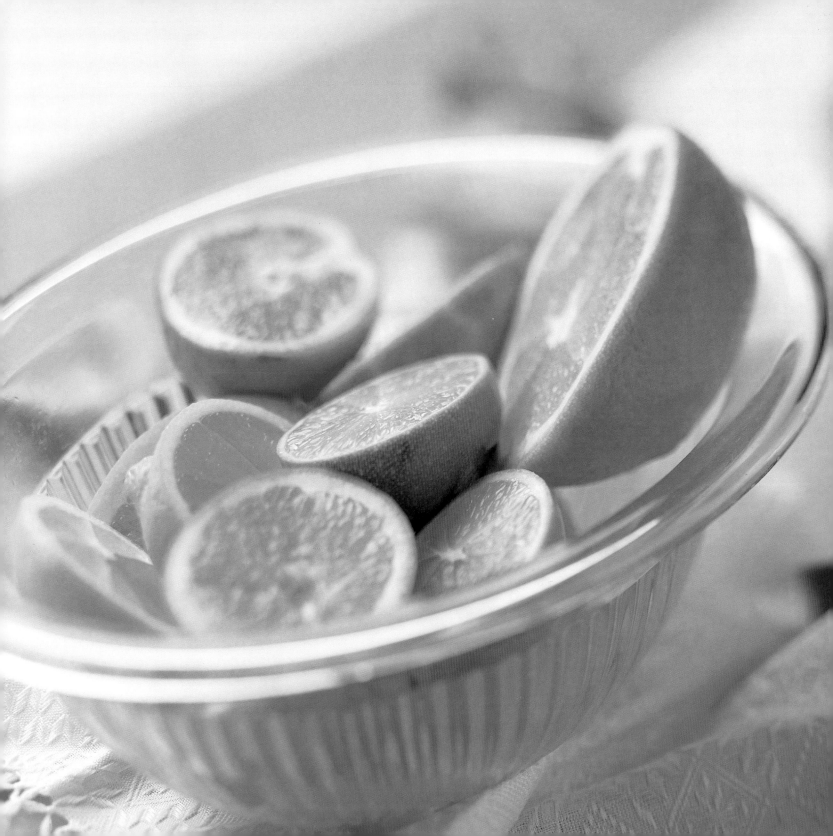

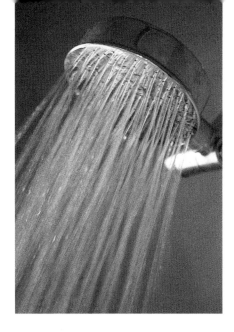

orange and ginger root cooler

This infusion will help calm your upset stomach and stimulate circulation. It can also be served warm to comfort you on a cold day.

3 cups of carbonated or spring water

1 tablespoon honey

2 oranges

2 inches fresh ginger root

Pour the carbonated water into a medium-sized pitcher, reserving ¼ cup. Pour the ¼ cup into a small bowl, add the honey, and stir until the honey dissolves.

Pour the dissolved honey and water into the pitcher. Slice one orange and add it to the pitcher. Add the juice from the other orange. Slice the ginger root very thin and add it to the pitcher. Allow the mixture to sit for 15 to 20 minutes. Pour over crushed ice in a glass and serve. Serves 2.

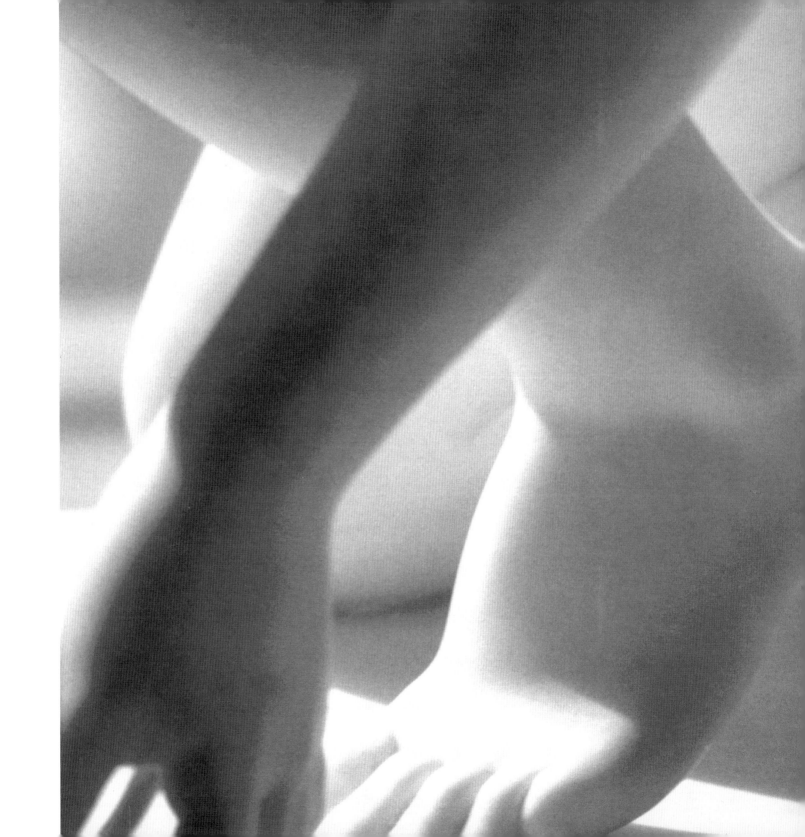

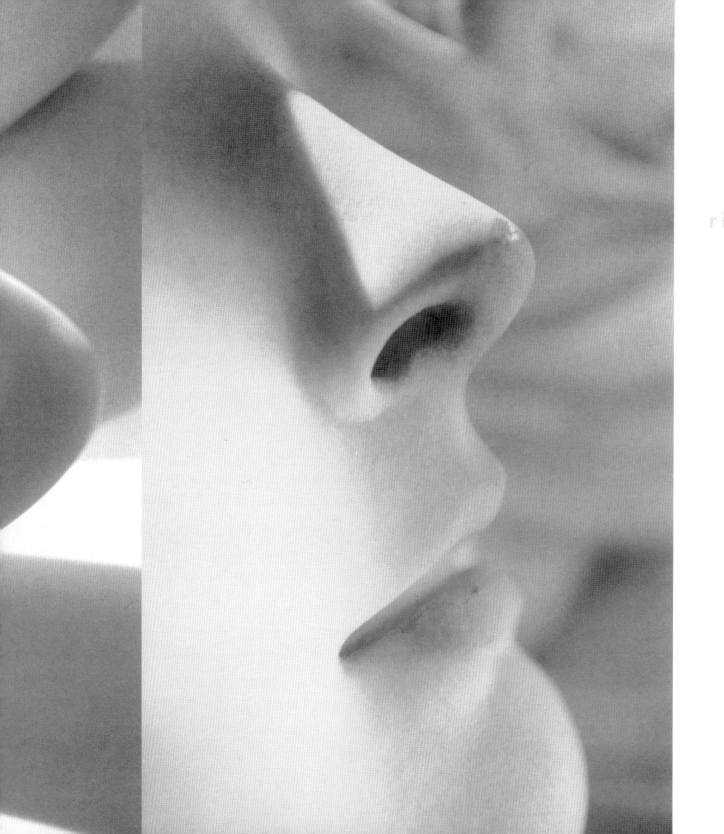

ritual

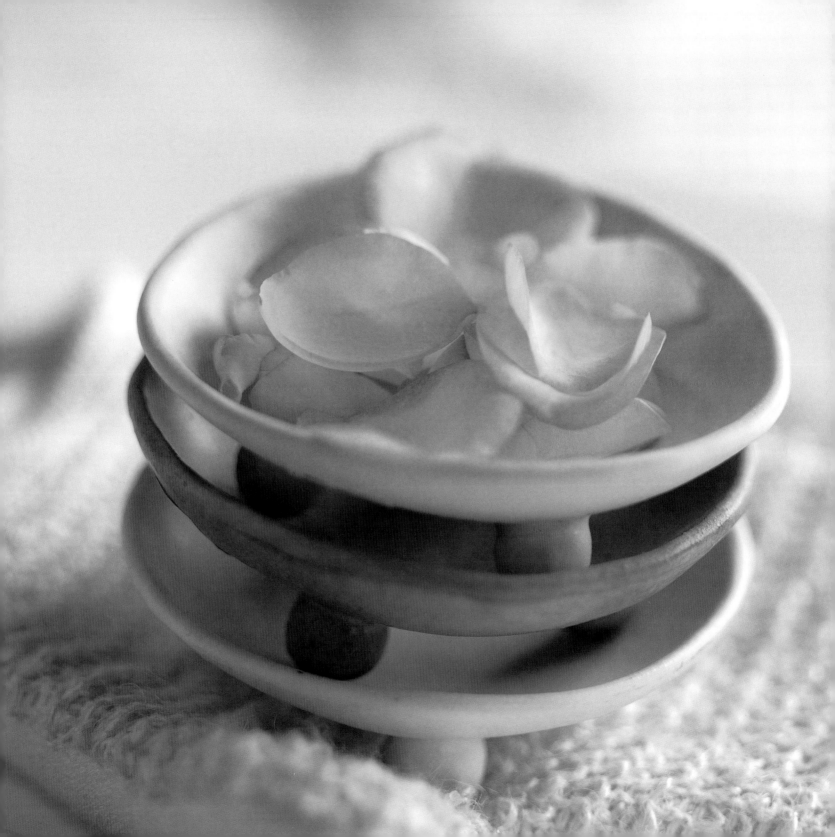

When she rises in the morning I linger to watch her;

Spreads the bath-cloth underneath the window

    And the sunbeams catch her

    Glistening white on the shoulders,

    While down her sides the mellow

    Golden shadow glows as

    She stoops to the sponge, and the swung breasts

    Sway like full blown yellow

    Gloire de Dijon roses.

She drips herself with water, and the shoulders

Glisten as silver, they crumple up

Like wet and falling roses, and I listen

For the sluicing of their rain-dishevelled petals.

    In the window full of sunlight

        Concentrates her golden shadow

    Fold on fold, until it glows as

    Mellow as the glory roses.

D. H. Lawrence

No doubt, Eden's residents took their showers beneath the pure cascade of a Garden waterfall. The wandering minstrel or peddler of an earlier era, waking in green mansions to a summer cloudburst, might well have stripped and showered in solitude there beneath accommodating trees. With the water rushing from the mouth of a stone panther or lion, the bathers of antiquity poured clean, cold water over themselves as the final step in a series of bodily cleansings.

Traditionally, Japanese bathers "shower" before their bath so they don't contaminate the bathwater with soap and grime. In the *sento*—the public bath—bathers sit on little stools before a spigot, energetically scrubbing themselves with a terry cloth washcloth and a bar of soap, lathering their bodies, and rinsing clean by dousing themselves with fresh water.

Nowadays, the morning shower has become nearly a universal ritual, with most Americans showering seven or more times a week. For many, the shower has proven either an adjunct or alternative to the morning cup of coffee. Outside of a spontaneous plunge into an alpine lake, there are few experiences as envigorating as a long, warm shower followed by a brief,

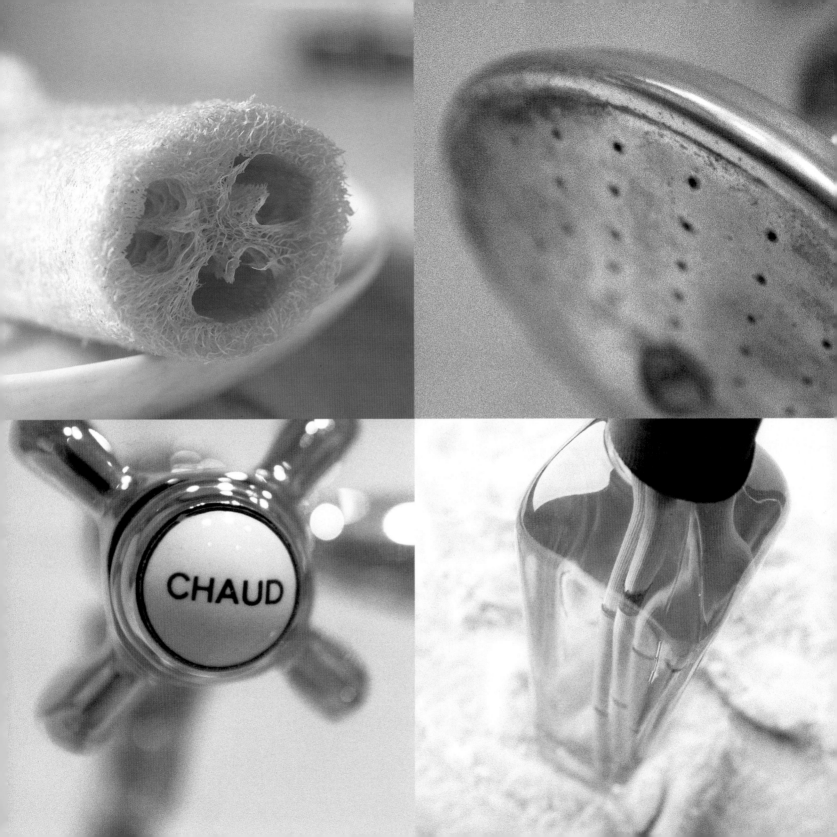

cool one. Standing, half-awake, head thrown back beneath the shower-head's steady spray, one moves effortlessly from sleepiness to vitality. The mind clears; the body glistens; and the spirit feels like singing.

benefits of bathing

Throughout the classical period, bathing was thought to promote general good health and longevity. Hippocrates, father of Western medicine, asserted that bathing could balance the humors and relieve ailments such as rheumatism and digestive disorders. Thermal baths were thought to promote respiration, relieve fatigue, and cure headaches while cold showers were used to relieve swelling and painful joints. By inducing sweating, a very warm bath was used to bring down a high fever. Practitioners of traditional Chinese medicine also recognized the positive effects of warm water and recommended that their patients drink warm to hot water to feed their "metabolic fire," what the Chinese call *yang chi*.

In the West, the medical benefits of bathing were forgotten during the Middle Ages, but the recovery of ancient medical texts during the Renaissance revived enthusiasm among the elites for the therapeutic bath.

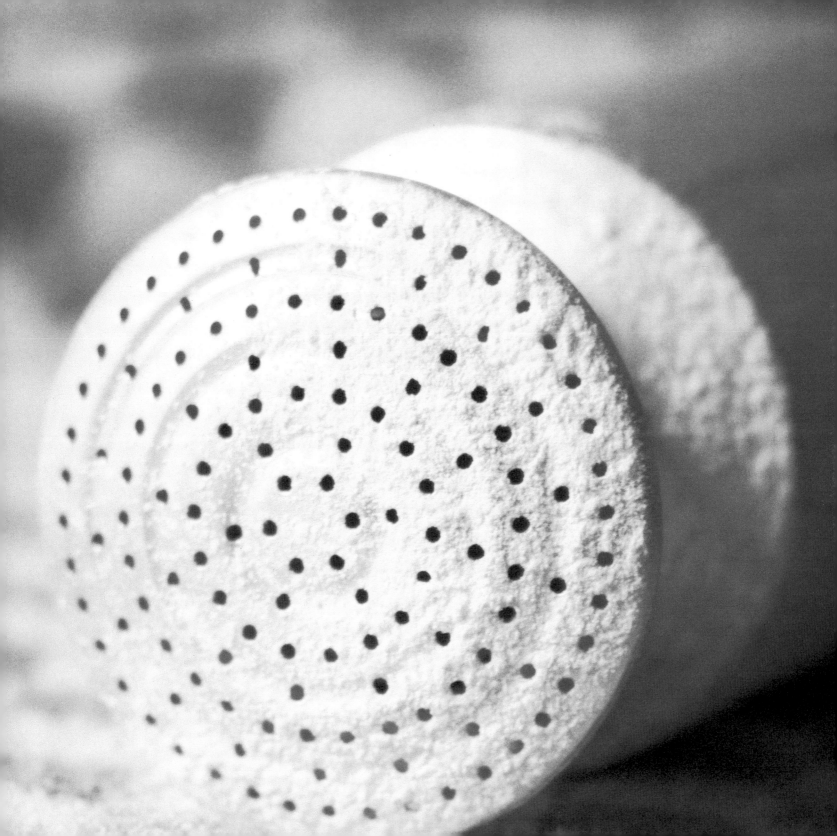

The spa was embraced by seventeenth-century France, Germany, and England—though the Church condemned the baths as hotbeds of sexual transgression. In an effort to take full advantage of water's healing properties, numerous Europeans imbibed, bathed, swam, and rinsed. Doctors and chemists undertook thorough analysis of the waters, convincing those who frequented the spas that the waters contained minerals that were effective against a myriad of illnesses. Charles Darwin, Charles Dickens, and Thomas Carlyle "took the cure" in the baths at Malvern, England, because the water was supposed to relieve disorders caused by severe intellectual exertions. And before the advent of modern drug therapy, it was common practice in many mental institutions to bathe patients in very warm water to make them more passive.

Today, luxury spas offer numerous treatments for relaxing our stress-weary bodies and minds. Mud baths, enzyme baths, salt scrubs, and seaweed body wraps are popular ways of detoxifying the body and softening the skin. The type of "mud" used by most American spas is a combination of volcanic ash and peat moss mixed with water from hot springs. With its heavy consistency, it at once envelopes and supports the body.

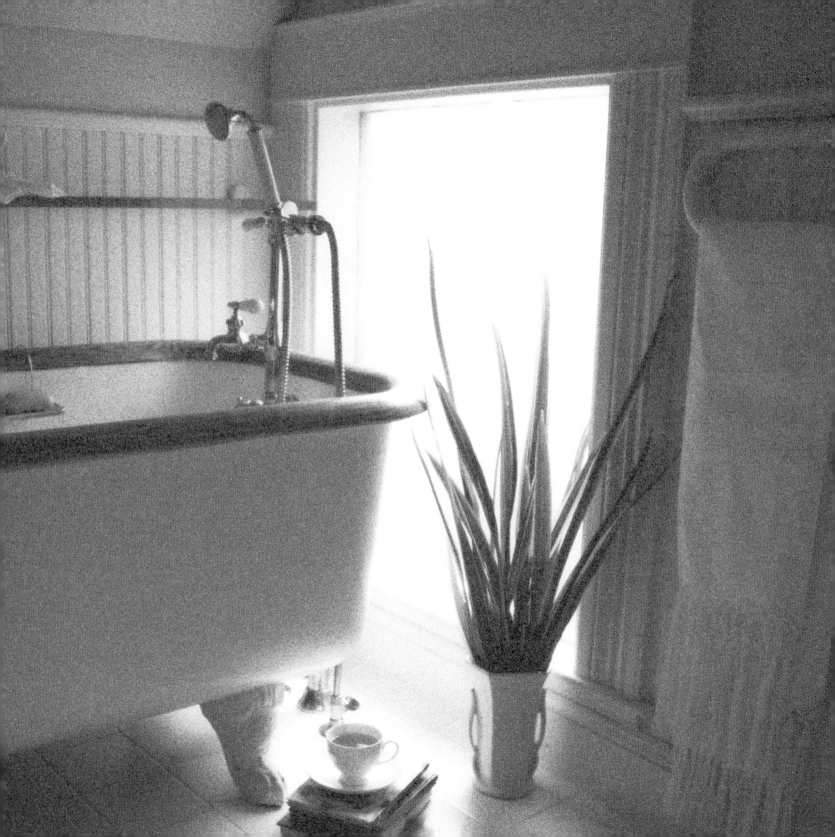

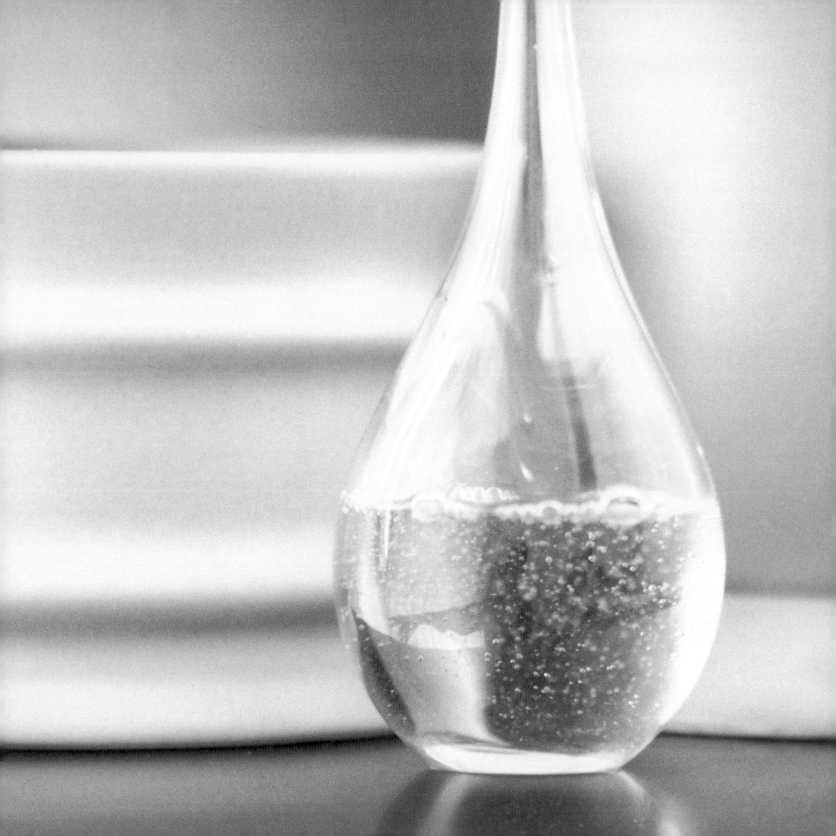

Japanese enzyme baths contain hundreds of active enzymes, which increase circulation, stimulate digestion, and smooth the skin. The fermenting enzymes give off bubbles that make the enzyme bath's heat much less intense than the mud bath's. Dry saunas and steam baths are also thought to be therapeutic for the overworked mind and body. Dry saunas descend from Scandinavian traditions; steam baths are related to the Turkish bath. Both cleanse the body by inducing perspiration, which removes toxins and increases circulation, improving one's energy.

What we call 'I'
is just a swinging door
which moves
when we inhale
and when we exhale.

Shunryu Suzuki

You need neither spa nor steam nor Turkish bath for any number of everyday bath therapies. The warmth and sublime pressure of the water encourages the body to relax and the skin to become softer, more permeable, and more sensitive. With herbs added to the water, either as a bundled infusion of whole herbs or as essential oils, a bath becomes a therapy for a variety of discomforts. Blended together for your morning bath, lavender, rosemary, eucalyptus, and ginger make a perfect decongestant remedy and cold fighter. Herbal baths can also offer headache relief, ease menstrual discomfort, or lessen varicose veins. Individual oils work gentle wonders, too: a few drops of rose petal oil can restore the skin's moisture balance, smooth wrinkles, and reduce redness.

Perhaps the most common impetus to soak in a bath is overexertion. After that first day back on the courts following a winter's hiatus, the body's complaints may be loud and clear. Fortunately, relief is just a hot bath away. Because warm water is penetrating and surrounding, a long soak with mineral or Epsom salts can be as soothing as a good massage.

Taking a bath before a chiropractic adjustment or deep tissue massage is also beneficial. Once again, the muscles relax making our bodies more receptive to both realignment and release. Bathing is also the recommended follow-up to many physical therapies. Be sure, whenever you take your bath, that you're truly comfortable, then lean back and get well.

aromatherapy

Aromatic essences are volatile, oily, fragrant botanical substances that can be obtained in a variety of ways. You can press flowers or herbs to release the oils into the water, pour boiling water on them to create an infusion, or make a decoction by boiling the herbs to create a strong potion. Or you can use oils with herb and flower extractions. You can tailor a bath to your mood and needs; it can be calming or stimulating, medicinal, or sensual.

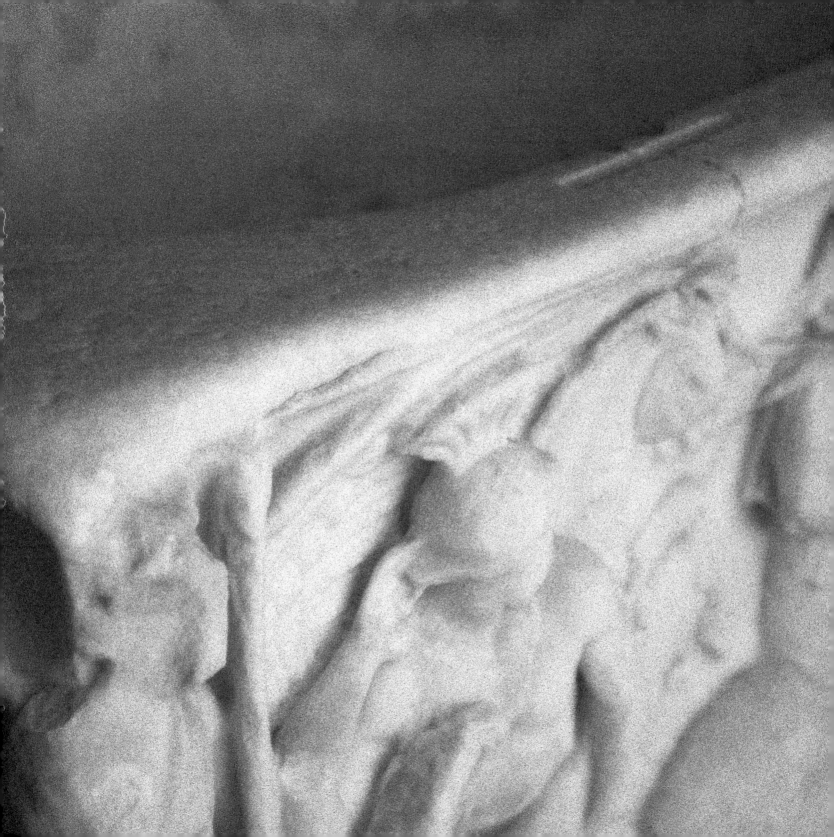

The Roman herbalist Pliny the Elder recommended baths of **chamomile** to relieve headaches and disorders of the kidneys, liver, and bladder. Steep chamomile flowers in boiling water for fifteen minutes, then pour into the bath. The flowers' oils are anti-inflammatory and antispasmodic, relieving skin disorders as well as menstrual cramps.

Pliny the Elder thought **mint** the loveliest of the herbs: "The very smell of it ," he said, "reanimates the spirit." Menthol gives the herb its smell and beneficial effects. In traditional Chinese medicine, mint is defined as a cooling herb. On a hot summer day, a tub of cool mint water will invigorate you, leaving your skin tingling. Soak crushed mint leaves in a bowl of water, strain, chill, and add to your bath.

The **rose** is queen of flowers, and the petals contain both an astringent and oils—the most precious is extracted from the damask roses that grow in Bulgaria. A perfumer might use 60,000 roses to procure one ounce of pure essential oil. A less costly version for the bath can be captured at home by soaking petals in vegetable oil. Or make rosewater by soaking bruised petals in water, then gently heating the mixture for a few minutes.

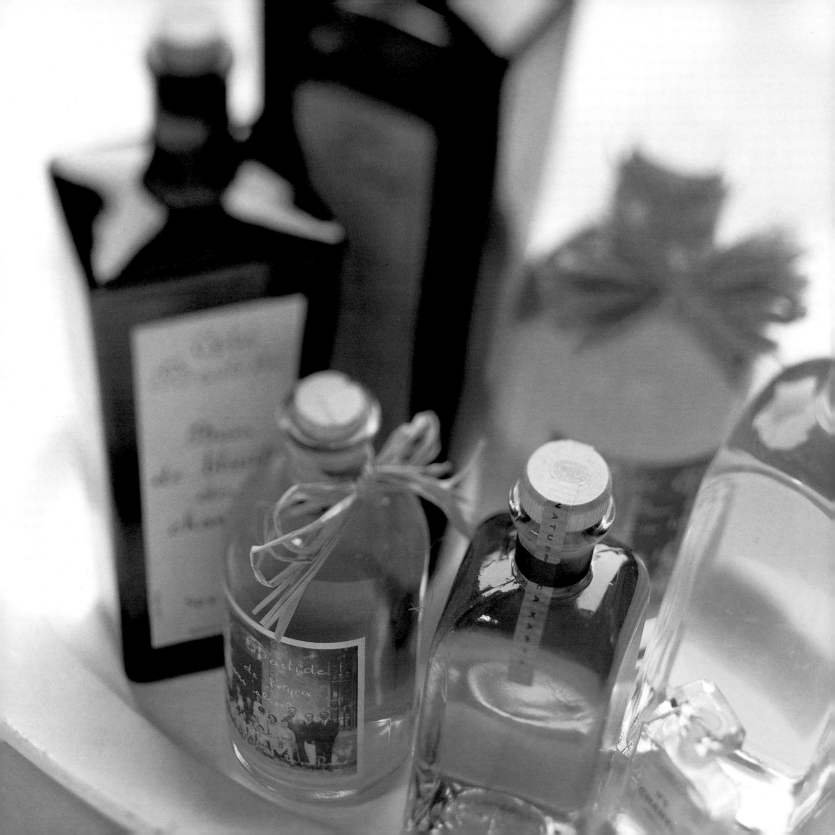

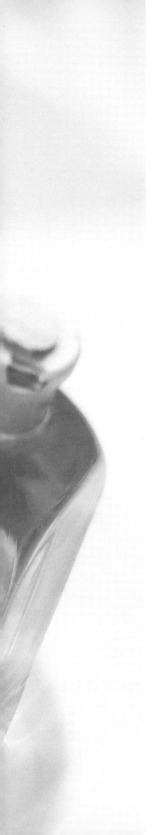

The Greeks believed that **rosemary** improved memory, inspiring students to wear garlands of the herb when they prepared for exams. A bath of rosemary has long been believed to be a cure for rheumatism, eczema, bruises, and wounds. The flowers and leaves contain a volatile oil that increases circulation. Make an infusion with the leaves and flowers, and add to your bathwater for a refreshing and stimulating experience.

The elegant tendril-like **ylang-ylang** flower blooms on the islands of Southeast Asia. Its sweet, heady fragrance is thought to be an aphrodisiac. Symbol of the honeymoon in Indonesia, its flowers are scattered over the bed of the wedding chamber. When steamed, ylang-ylang flowers release a captivating essence. Ylang-ylang is believed to soothe an accelerated breathing rate or abnormally rapid heartbeat.

A tablespoon of **seaweed**-enriched liquid from your local health food store can be added to your bath to remove toxins such as uric acid and excess sulfates by raising the body temperature and encouraging perspiration. Seaweed is naturally rich in magnesium, zinc, iron, iodine, and sodium, and has become increasingly popular for spa massages and wraps.

the turkish bath

The Turkish Bath has long been romanticized by travelers to the Middle East. In the early eighteenth century, Lady Mary Wortley Montagu was the first Western woman to penetrate the magical realm of the women's *ham-mam,* the public bath, and in her letters she describes their magnificence: "To see so many fine women naked, in different postures, some in conversation, some working, others drinking coffee or sherbet, and many negligently lying on their cushions, while their slaves (generally pretty girls of seventeen or eighteen) are employed in braiding their hair in several pretty fancies. In short, it's the women's coffeehouse, where all the news of the town is told, scandal invented, etc.—they generally take this diversion once a week, and stay there at least four or five hours."

All morning you've lain
in the blessing
of this cloudy room,
barely aware
of the blurred gestures
of others—one washing,
one setting down a cup—
the steam a wish
for wealth or love.

In this ancient place,
this splendid display
of marble and geometry,
it is ordinary
to leave the world behind.

And here your life turns,
unnoticed,
like the Earth
on its axis

as an old song,
seeps through the walls—
O kirmiizi, O beyaz gul,
O white, O red rose—
and stands in
for everything unreachable
reached.

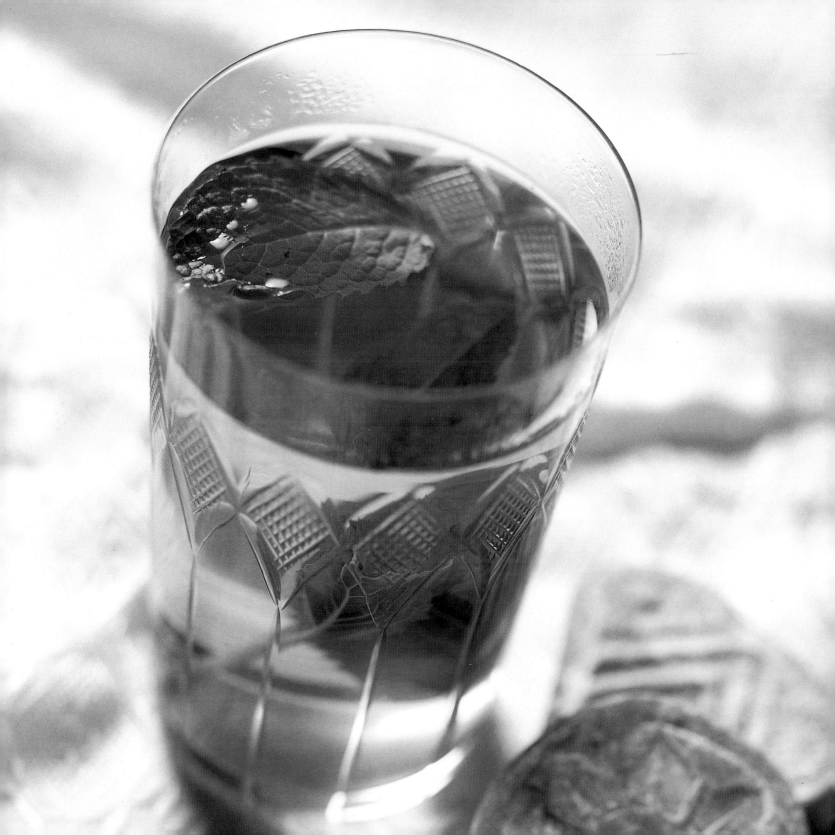

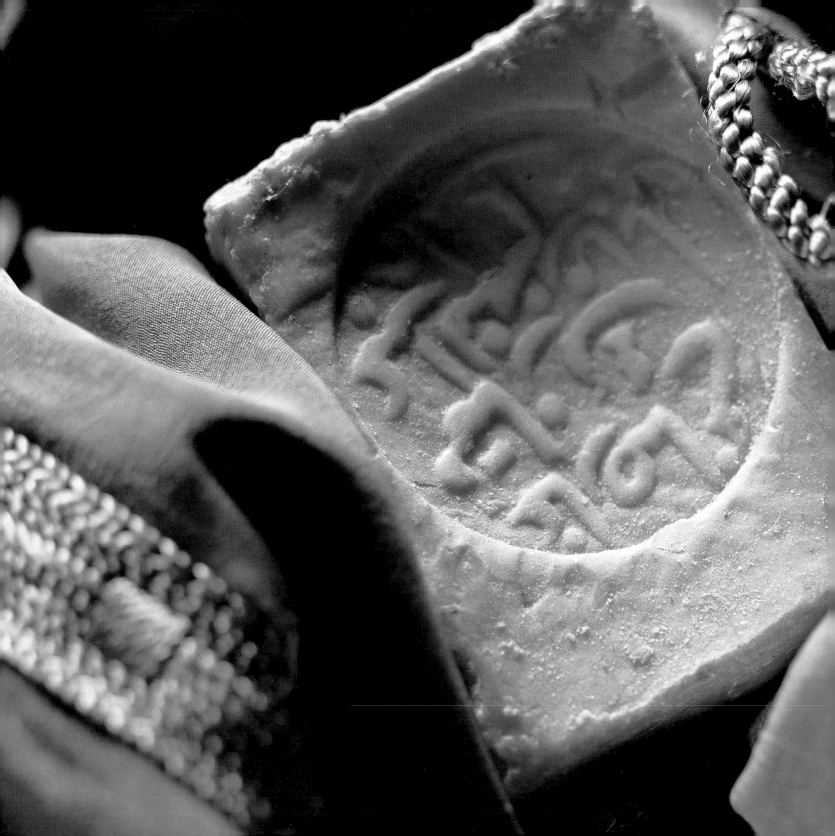

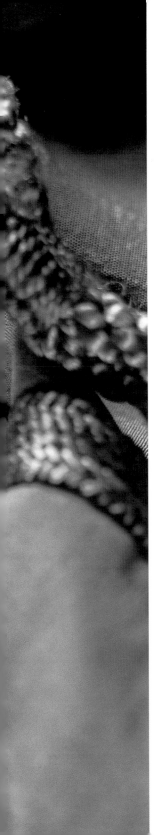

Even today, when homes have private baths, the women of Damascus and Istanbul go to the baths to relax and gossip in this steamy atmosphere. The Turkish bath is the direct descendent of the Roman bath; however, the drier desert climes of the Middle East do not make Romanesque pools of running water very practical. So Turkish bathers cleanse by perspiring and then dousing themselves to remove dirt and dead skin.

Classically inspired, the architecture of the Turkish bath is always distinguished and elegant, with high vaulted ceilings, rich marble veneers, stained-glass skylights, and fountains embellished with geometric designs. Women going to spend a day at the baths pack special hammam food in steel tins—lentils and rice cooked with cinnamon, perhaps, or sliced cucumber salad with dill. In the bath, the women wrap themselves in fine cotton sateen and wear wooden clogs to protect their feet from the hot, slick marble floors. After several hours of perspiring, scrubbing, lathering, and rinsing, a woman enshrouds herself with three thick towels—one around the torso, one about the shoulders, and one on the head like a turban. She then retires to a chamber decorated with colorful, hand-woven rugs and Damascene pillows to sip sweet mint tea or fresh strawberry juice.

the finnish bath

The sauna's simplest form is a room built of logs that contains a large stove piled with stones. When a Scandinavian sets out to build a new home, he begins with the sauna. The Saturday afternoon sauna is an age-old Scandinavian tradition. Early in the morning, the firebox is stoked and lit so that by evening the stones are red-hot and the room is between 190 and 200 degrees Fahrenheit.

The Scandinavians believe that taking a sauna is more than a means of getting clean: It's a way to relax and enjoy the company of friends and neighbors. It's just as customary to invite a guest for a sauna as for dinner. The Finns say, "Two places are holy—the church and the sauna." In the sauna, one should follow the same quiet, reserved etiquette that one does in church. Singing and talking should be kept to a minimum, and whistling is a definite violation of the sauna's sanctity.

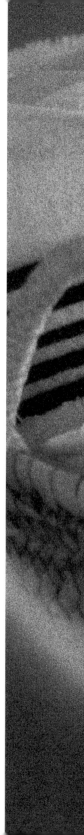

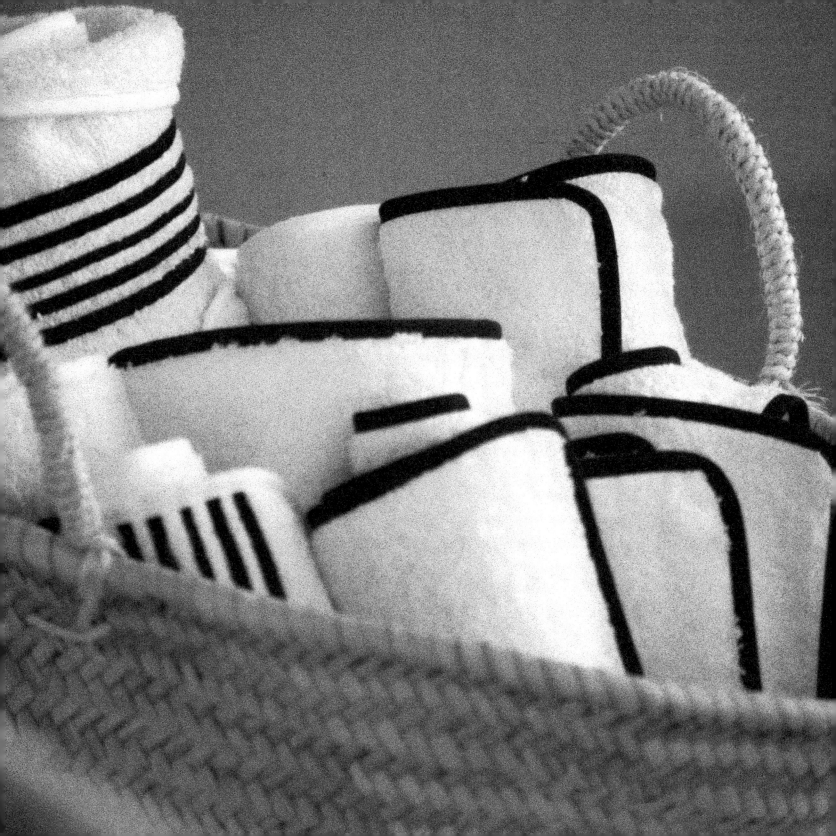

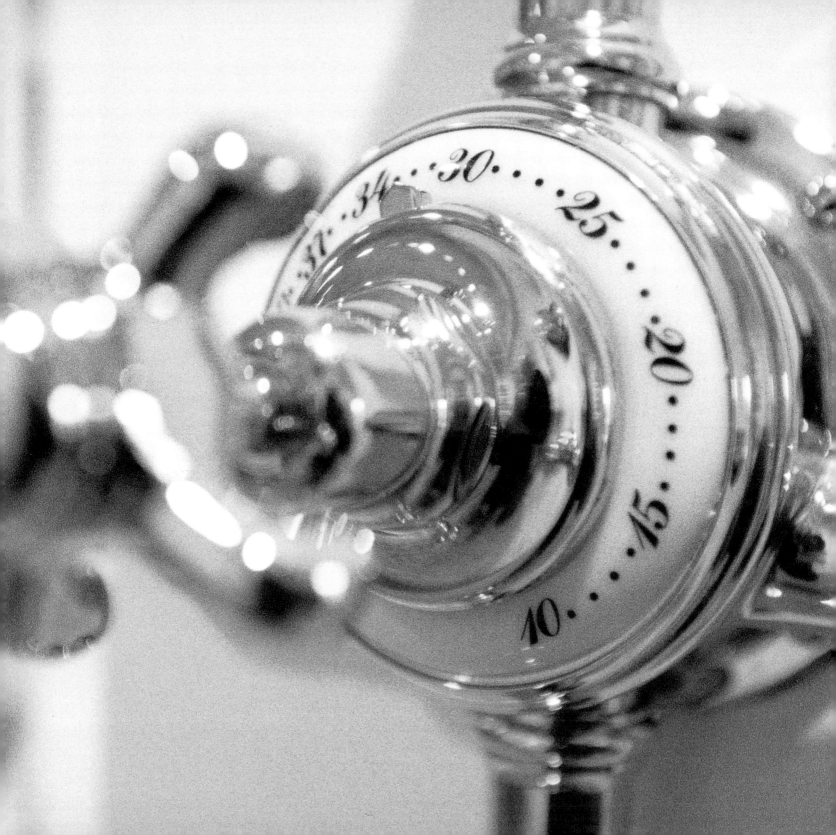

The ritual begins by sitting in the dry heat to start the flow of perspiration. To increase the heat's intensity the bather "makes steam" by throwing water on the hot rocks, of which it's said, "One dipper for each man, and one for the sauna." After about twenty minutes, one should cool off with a shower, or by jumping into a nearby lake, or by rolling in the snow—without a doubt the most exhilarating of the three. Another important component of the ritual is brushing the body with a birch whisk. Leafy branches from the curly or silver birch are gathered in early summer and bound together. To increase circulation, one whisks the body from top to bottom. Then one soaps up. It's quite pleasant to whip up a lather with a birch whisk; the fragrance of birch lingers on the skin. After rinsing off, a bather may enjoy another or several more rounds of heating up and cooling off.

Everywhere in many lands gush forth
        beneficent waters, here cold,
there hot, there both...
        promising relief to the sick...

Pliny the Elder

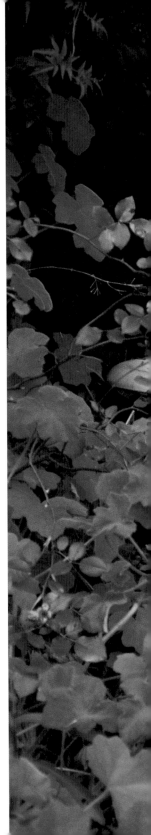

a traveler's notes: outdoor baths

There was the one on a deck in Mendocino, a sitzbath painted yellow by the morning light streaming through branches of hillside oak and madrone. Then, there was the one in the mountains of Bali, high above the rice paddies—in fresh spring water funneled through an ancient pipe into a crystalline pool surrounded by orchids and spires of grass. And, years later, on a Paiute reservation in Nevada, in jerryrigged pools where the locals had managed to harness the hot, sulfurous geyser at the north end of Pyramid Lake—a last vestige of the continent's antediluvian seas, teeming with cutthroat trout and ringed with cathedralesque tufas.

In the Emirates, just inland from the Straights of Hormuz—the bottleneck through which the Persian Gulf flows into the Indian Ocean—a bedouin pointed the way to a place in the lunar landscape of the coastal mountains, a pool formed by a subterranean river that surfaced briefly, for just a few kilometers. It was magic, that oasis with sweet water: bunches of date palms, and tulle grass—all vermilion—studded with dragonflies. And above them all, one constant beauty—the sky: vast, still, sheltering.

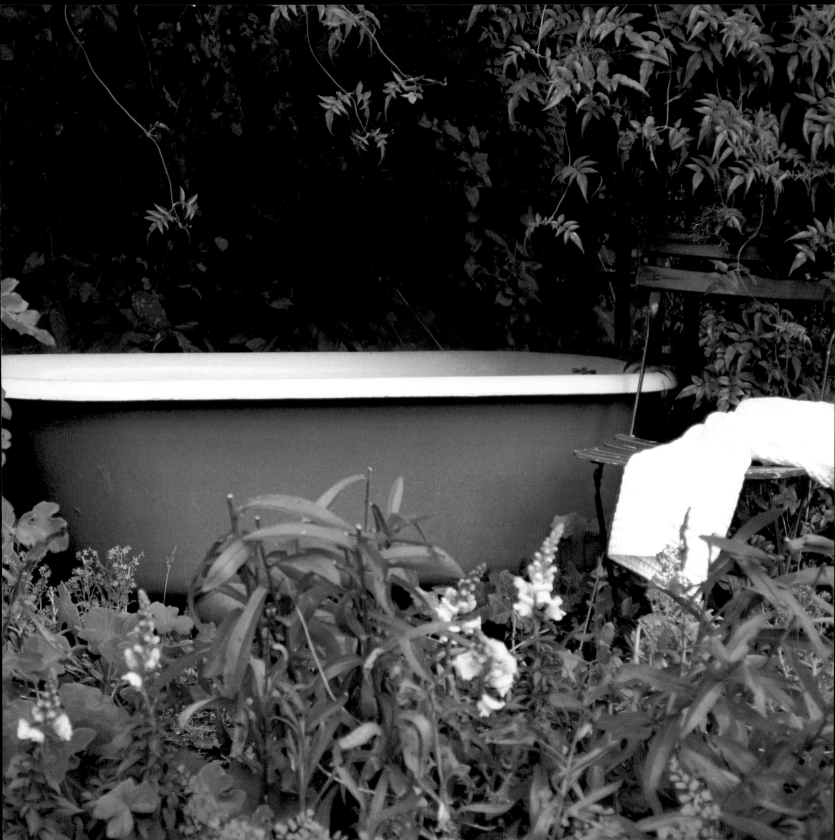

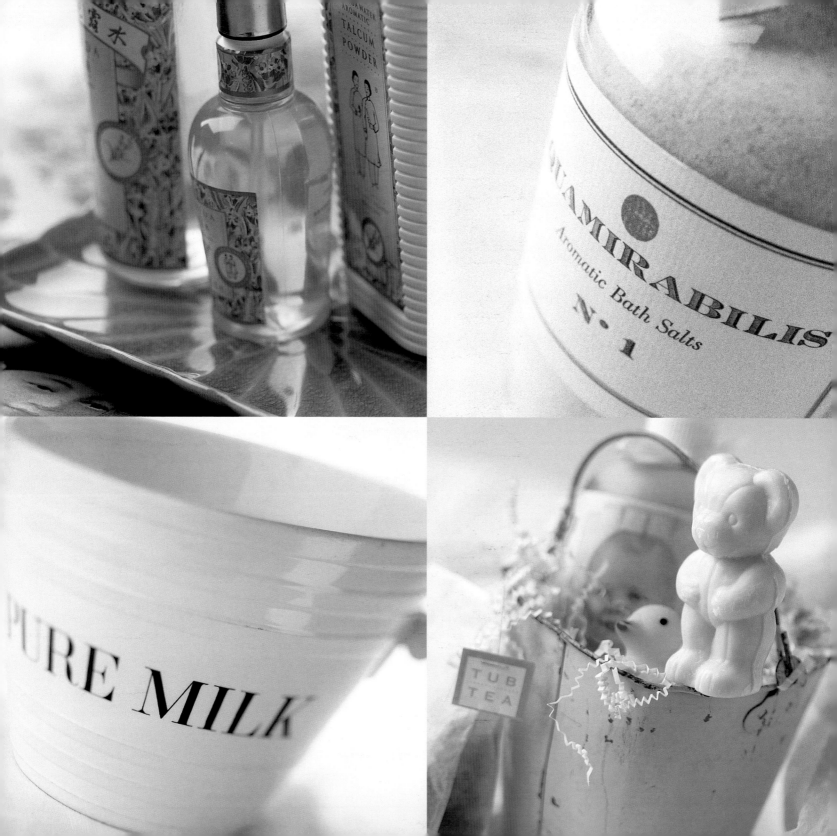

TALCUM POWDER

MIRABILIS

Aromatic Bath Salts

N. 1

PURE MILK

TUB TEA

bathing in luxury

The Bubble Bath   A hundred million bubbles—one long, soothing sound like the inscrutable rhythm of sand shifting on the ocean's floor. Now, this is luxury—white clouds perfumed with notes of lavender or peach. One scoops up a bounty of this white ethereality, making a generous crown.

The Milk Bath   Three young girls, each prettier than the other, lean over a scallop of marble and pour the star-white contents of three painted vessels into their queen's bath. She, Cleopatra, luxuriates there, submerged in a pool of the freshest milk and honey—all to prepare herself for her historic seduction of Marc Antony, her skin so soft he would compare it to the petals of the jasmine blossom.

Fantasy Bath   One: Three actors (the wild one, the rebel without a cause, and the enigmatic starlet) once filled a tub with champagne, the ultimate gesture of decadence. Two: On an ordinary tropical day, a Polynesian prince drew his lover's bath with cool water, setting three dozen gardenias afloat. Three: San Francisco, the Summer of Love, a tub full of cherry Jello and a couple of flower children (no marshmallows).

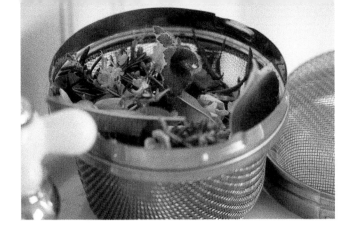

mesh ball infusions

Big mesh bath infusers are perfect containers for combining a variety of fresh ingredients and infusing your bath with the scents and soothing, relaxing, or invigorating properties of herbs and flowers. Hang the ball from your faucet in the path of flowing water, and reap the benefits.

for a rainy day

Soak in the tub and listen to the rain drops.

Handful of pine needles or juniper sprigs

3 broken cinnamon sticks

10 or so whole cloves

3 thick slices of fresh ginger

summer afternoon bath

A perfect finish to a balmy day.

2 sprigs pineapple mint

2 sprigs sage

Peel of one orange

Peel of one lime

Handful of lemon verbena leaves

spring morning

This crisp and naturally astringent bath is great if you're feeling a cold coming on. It is also a luxurious treat when healthy.

Large handful of eucalyptus leaves, torn

6 to 8 thick slices of ginger

Juice of one lemon, squeezed into bath

Few drops of neroli, the scent of

orange blossoms

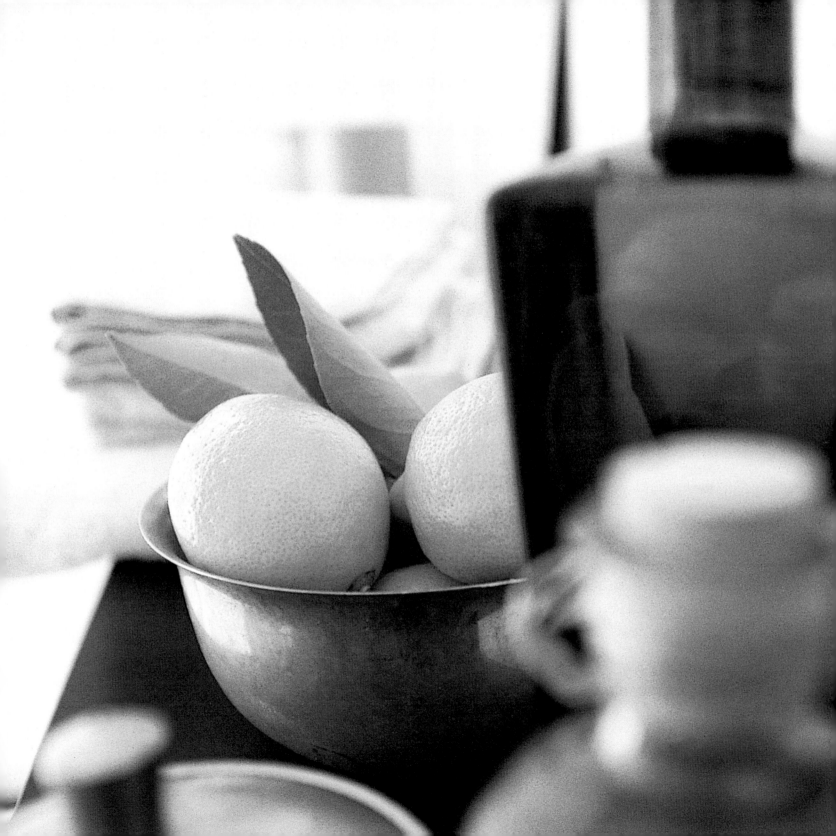

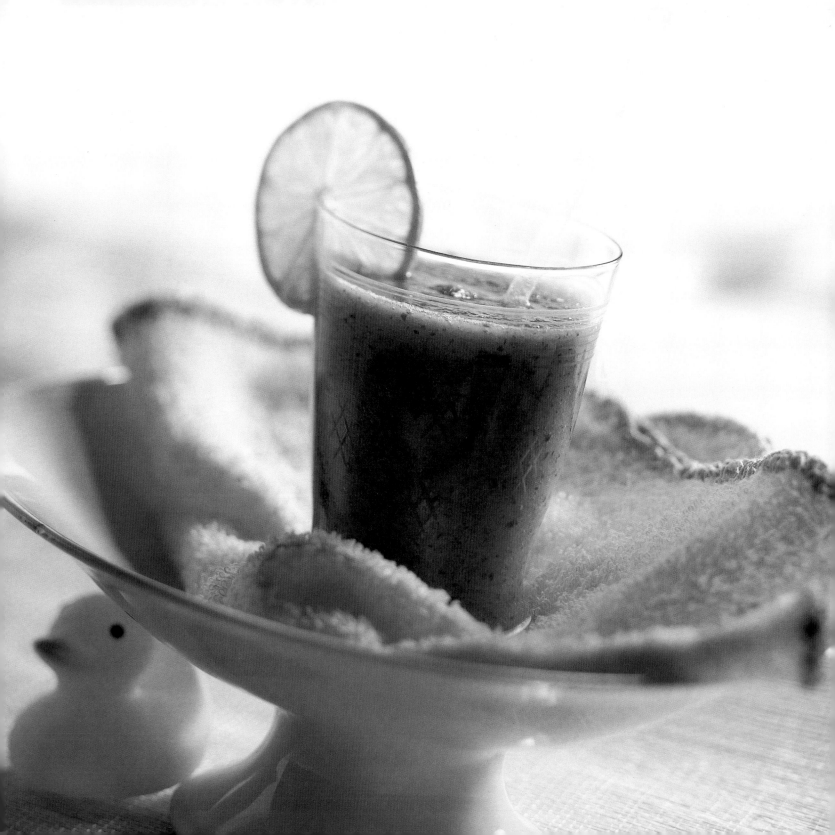

green blend

This is a cleansing and cooling blend. Both cucumber and melon draw out toxins while helping you maintain an inner coolness during a warm bath.

½ small honeydew melon, seeded

½ English cucumber, peeled and sliced

small handful of mint leaves, stems removed

juice from one lime

1 lime sliced for garnish

Scoop honeydew from rind and place it in a blender. Puree until smooth. Place cucumber, mint, and lime juice in blender and puree mixture for 10 to 15 seconds more. Serve in tall frozen glasses with lime slices. Serves 2 to 4.

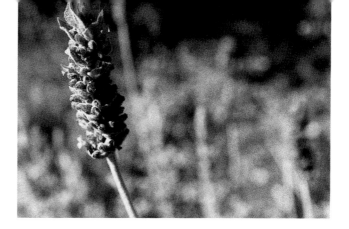

sweet and fragrant tea

This is a simple tisane of soothing chamomile and aromatic lavender blossom.

1 ¼ cups water

1 teaspoon dried chamomile

½ teaspoon dried lavender

1 sprig fresh lavender blossom (optional)

1 to 2 teaspoons honey

Bring the water to a boil. Place dried chamomile and lavender in a small wire-mesh teaball. Place the teaball and fresh lavender blossom in a teacup or mug and pour in boiling water. Stir in honey and allow tea to steep for 3 minutes before drinking. Serves 1.

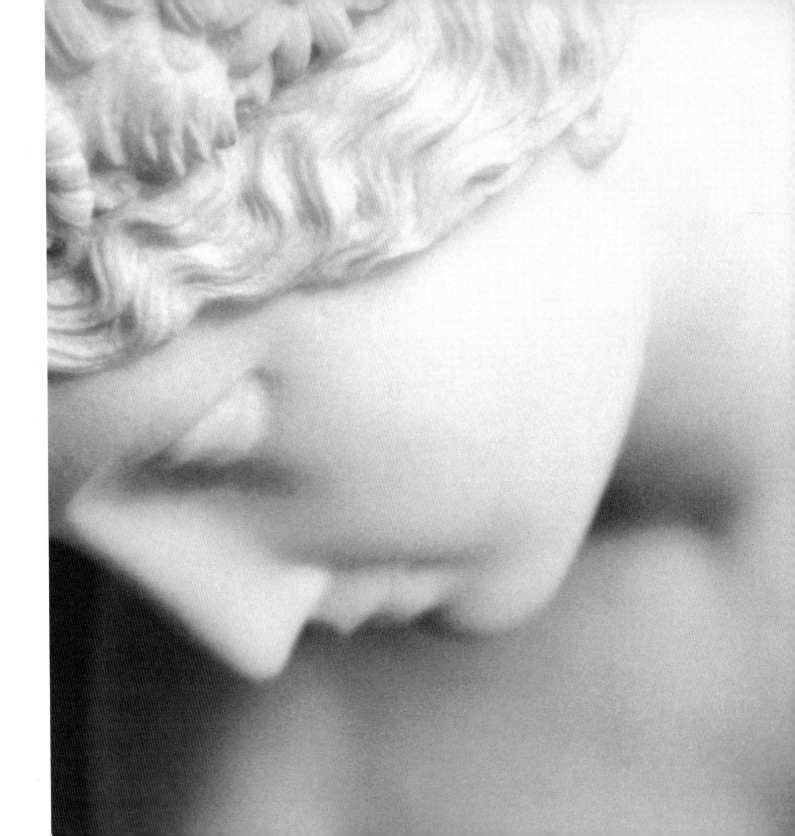

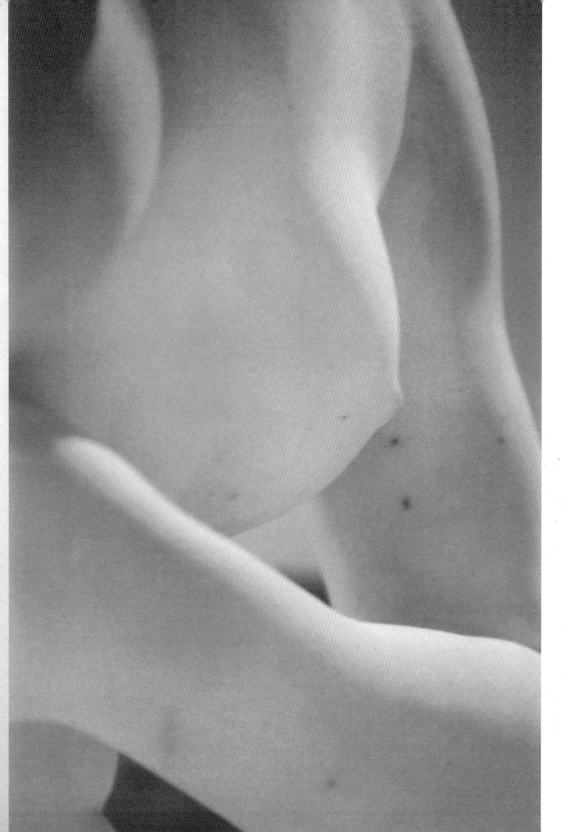

spirit

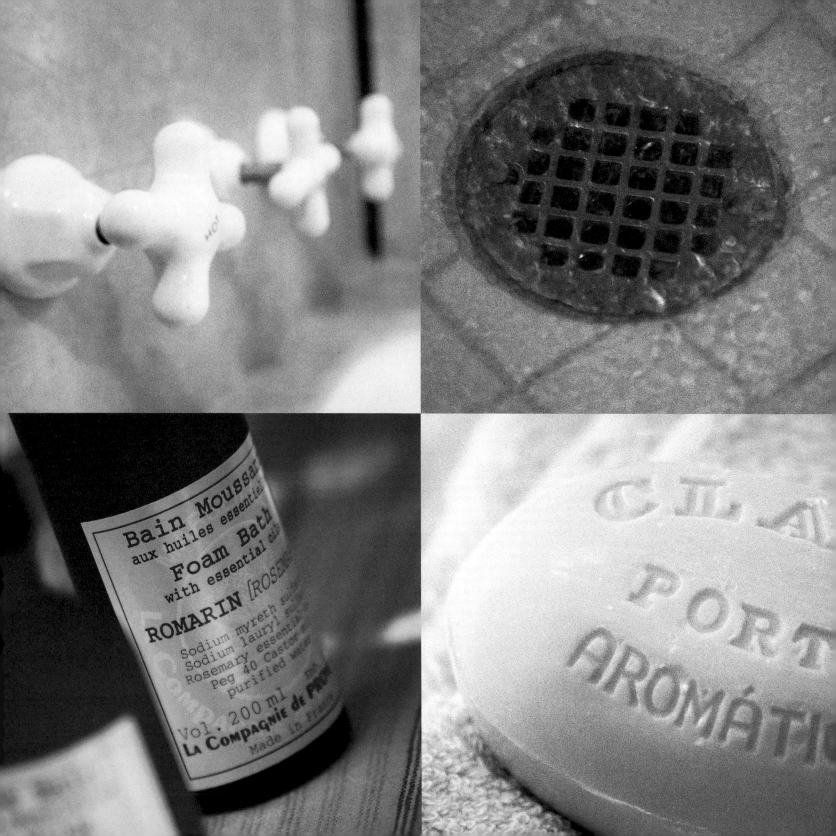

She went to the drawer

where she kept dozens of votives in case of a storm

and brought them all into the bathroom,

drew herself a bath and lit every candle—

their flames tipsy with steam.

And squinting just a little,

she found herself in that place by the sea where she'd slept

       through the rain in the beach grass,

       the fishermen going out before dawn,

       the horizon studded with the

       lights of boats from years ago.

In late October when we turn our clocks for fall, the morning light can

seem as fragile as those last moments of sleep when dream life and wak-

ing life merge, and like the Chinese sage, you cannot tell if you are the

proverbial butterfly dreaming you are the man or the man dreaming you

are the butterfly. Slip into a bath in this half-awake state, in this half light,

this dawn light so pale and delicate on porcelain, tiles, towels, straw mat.

Echoes of honey, oranges, a single red maple—the sun going down just as

you ease yourself down into bath water at the end of a long summer day.

The last rays of light come in from the world beyond the hills to this quiet

world you've made—where you sit, wash, and rest.

Each Bird Walking

Not while, but long after he had told me, I thought of him, washing his mother,

his bending over the bed and taking back the covers. There was a basin of water

and he dipped a washrag in and out of the basin, the rag

dripping a little onto the sheet as he turned from the bedside to the nightstand

and back... He turned her on her stomach and washed the blades of her shoulders,

the small of her back. "That's good," she said, "that's enough."   Tess Gallagher

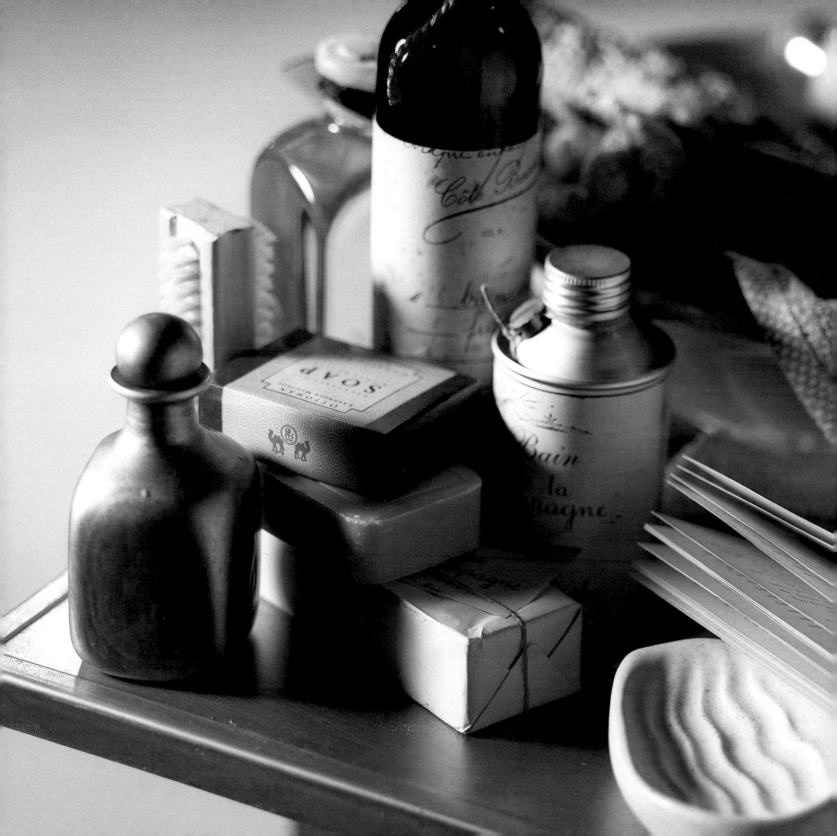

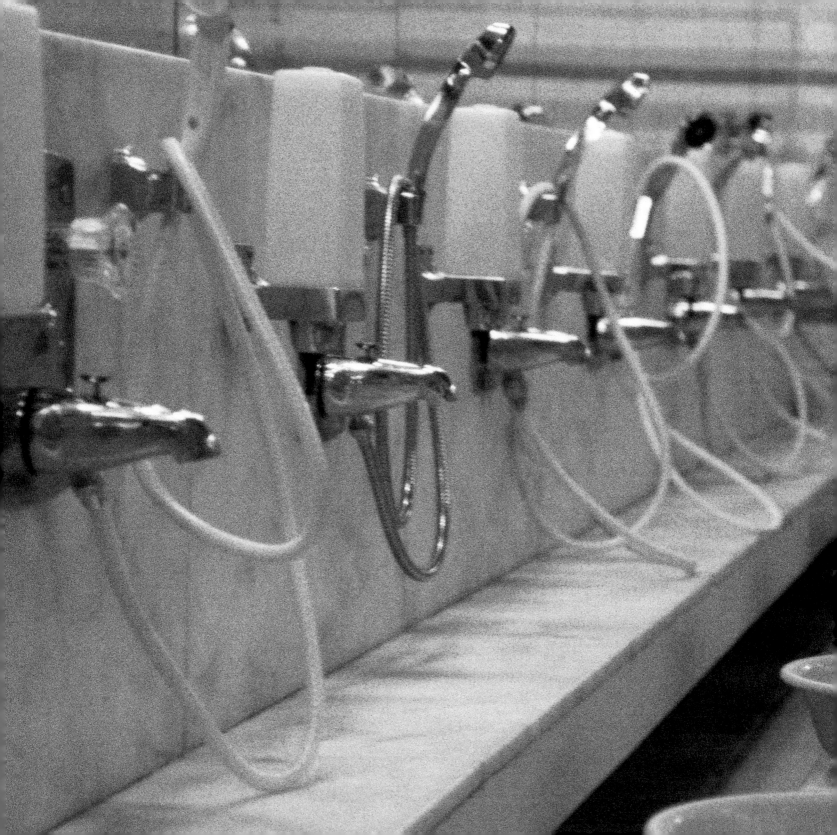

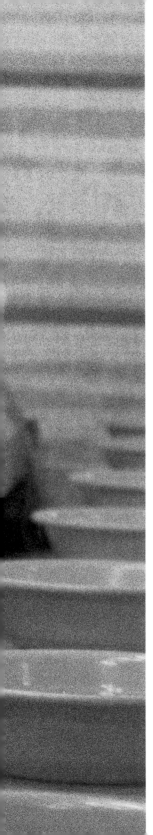

bathing in japan

A venerable claw-foot tub filled with steaming water. Your every cell buoyant, no longer limited by this world's gravity, you float inward, into the jeweled cord that is the ebb and flow of the universe. Lost in the water's gentle lapping at the edge of your porcelain sea, you remember the story of the Japanese empress who, it is said, vowed to bathe a thousand beggars with her own hands. And when the thousandth, a leper, stepped before her, she bathed him with the same loving kindness that she had the others. That leper, unbeknownst to her, was the Buddha.

In Japan, bathing has always been an act that transcends its utility. For the Japanese the process of bathing is a ceremony, a ritual that takes the bather to the spirit by way of the body. Whether bathing communally or alone, the Japanese bather washes before getting into the bath. Soaping up, rubbing down, and using a small bucket to rinse, one not only washes away the world's dust, but prepares the mind for a deeper cleansing—the bath that follows. The warm bathwater calms both body and mind, bringing about a languid ease, and daily concerns fall away. A man soaking in a *rotenburo*— a large open-air hot spring—listens to the rustling leaves overhead; a girl in a tile bathroom watches the steam rising. Such is tranquillity.

In Japan, bathing has always been considered a vital necessity. Fuel was allocated to heat water for bathing before being used for cooking or heating, though, for the most part, the multitude of hot springs on this volcanic island provided an abundant source of hot water. Many Shinto (the ancestral and regional traditions found throughout Japan) shrines, though they celebrate the mythological ancestors of powerful families, were actually established at springs and wells to guard community water supplies. The rites of *harai* (exorcism and purification) and *misogi* (ritual cleansing), ever present in Shinto ceremonies, in all likelihood were simply practical ways to keep the wells and springs clean for bathing, drinking, and cooking.

In the earliest Shinto myths, bathing is portrayed as a seminal act. Evil and immorality are closely associated with filth and impurity, whereas virtue and goodness follow from cleanliness. Legend has it that when Izanagi, the ultimate Shinto creator ancestor, washed his body, the other cosmic gods— the Sun, Moon, and Fertility—were born out of his bath. In his book *Meeting with Japan*, Fasco Maraini writes about the relationship of Shinto traditions and bathing: The bath is a domestic aspect of ancient

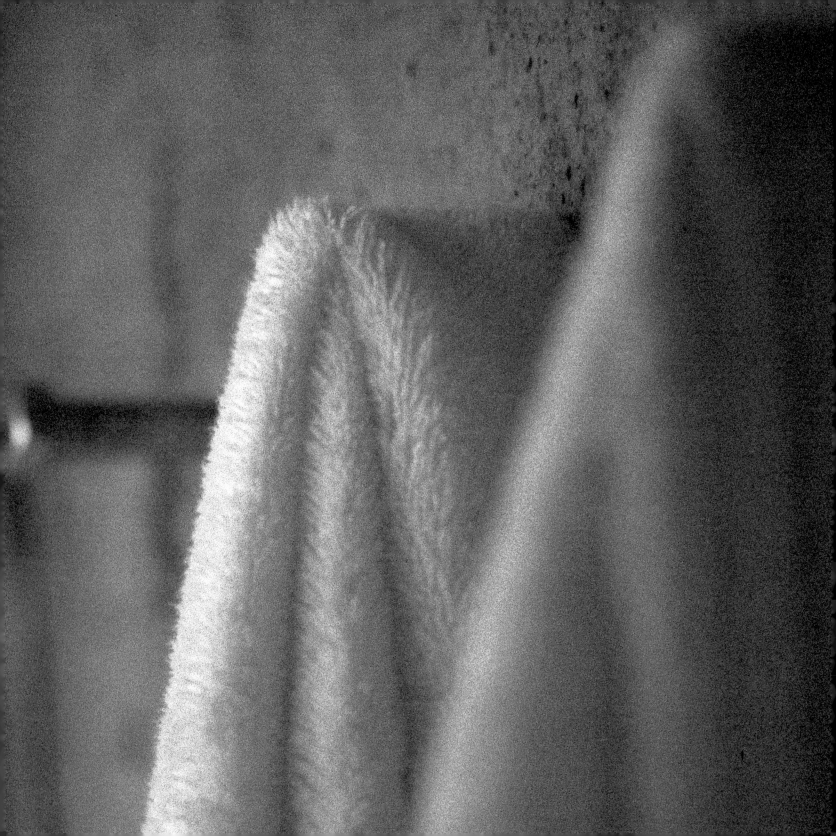

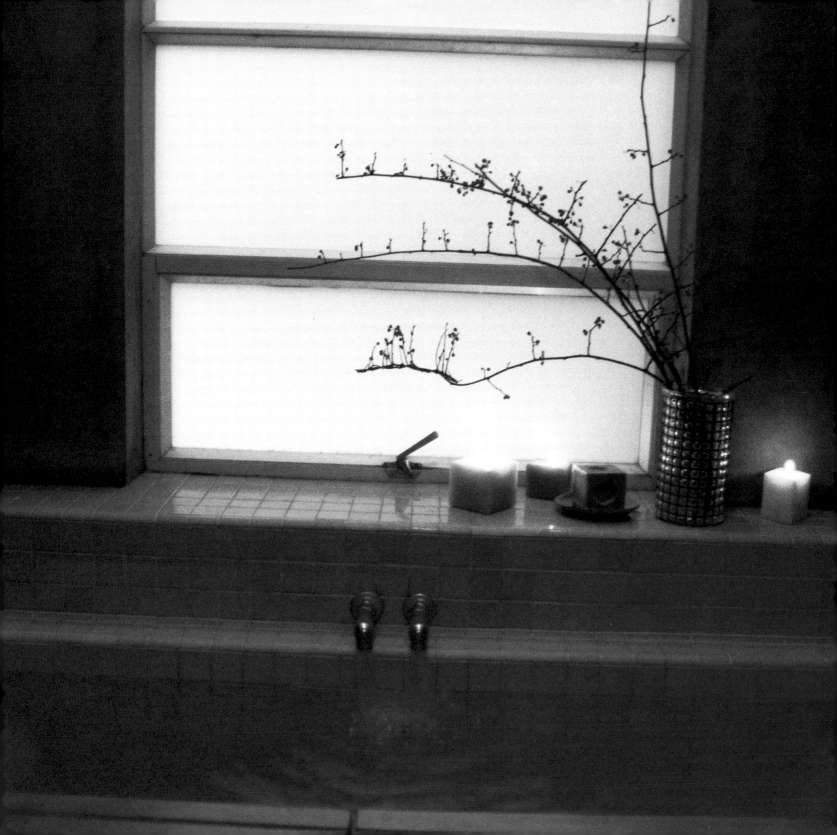

purification rites, which from the earliest times were an essential element of the Shinto cult. Every expression of religious feeling is a joyful thing: When man feels, however indirectly or remotely from his consciousness, that he is in harmony with God, with the gods, the invisible, he is happy, at peace with himself and others.

The Japanese believe that bathing is best when enjoyed with companions. Though most families in Japan have their own private baths, many still frequent the *sento* for a sense of community. And while the rattle of soap and scrub brushes in bath buckets and the clacking of wooden clogs is heard much less often now than in the past, the communal bath remains an affirmation of personal bonds, closeness, and kinship. *Hadaka no tsuki-ai*—"companions in nudity"—friends who bathe together—these friends are the closest of all.

"The old pond—

a frog jumps in,

sound of water."

Bashō

transforming the bath

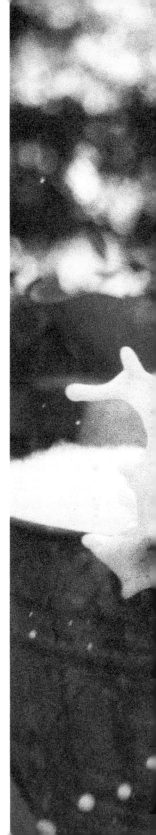

Giving Over   When you give a baby a bath you come to know him at his softest, glistening, and weightless. Like a cloud he floats, a tiny, bright-eyed angel. It's a time for you and him to talk—with your eyes and watery sounds. And you support him wholly, give him all of yourself as he gives over more and more, so pleased with himself, emerging—a little duck with a little stylish crest.

Giving Back   Going slowly, moving with love, tenderly shifting the limbs, washing them patiently—giving back. A creamy soap, a thick robe, a gentle touch. Giving an elder a bath can be a time for deep renewal, for renewing our relationship with someone dear to our hearts, by making the ritual purely an opportunity to give back.

Giving In   Some dogs seem to have it all: trendy collars, down-filled beds, organic pet food. Our's *does*—because she has her own personal outdoor, hot-water shower. Not that she relishes bath time, but she does stand for it—quite literally—stands there like some kind of canine arrow with her nose pointing in one direction and her heart in another, soaking up all our affection as we lather her with coconut oil soap and never-ending praise.

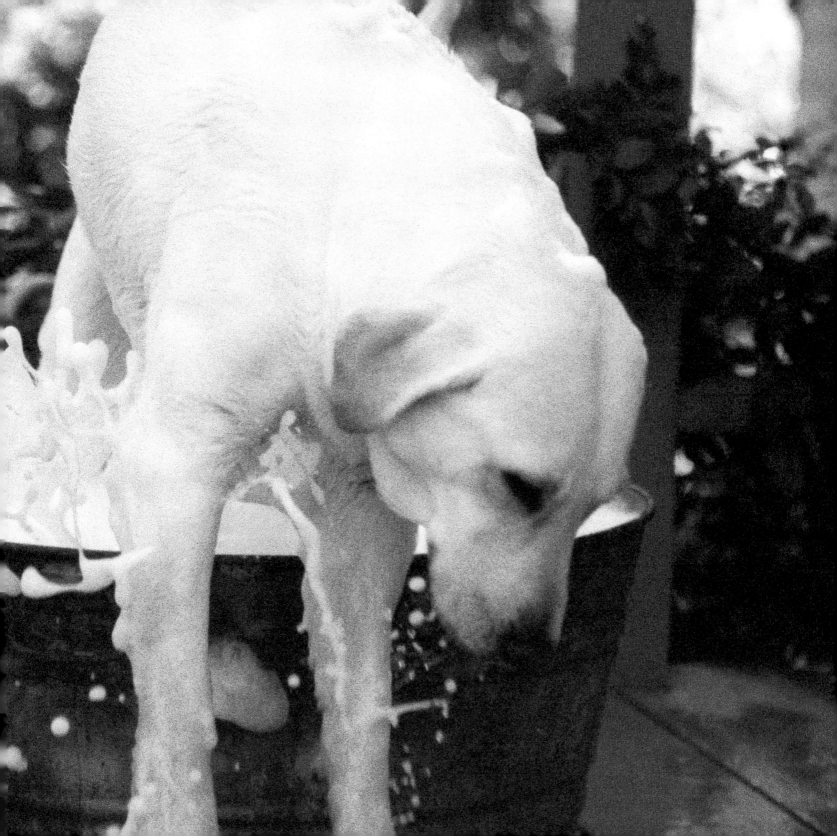

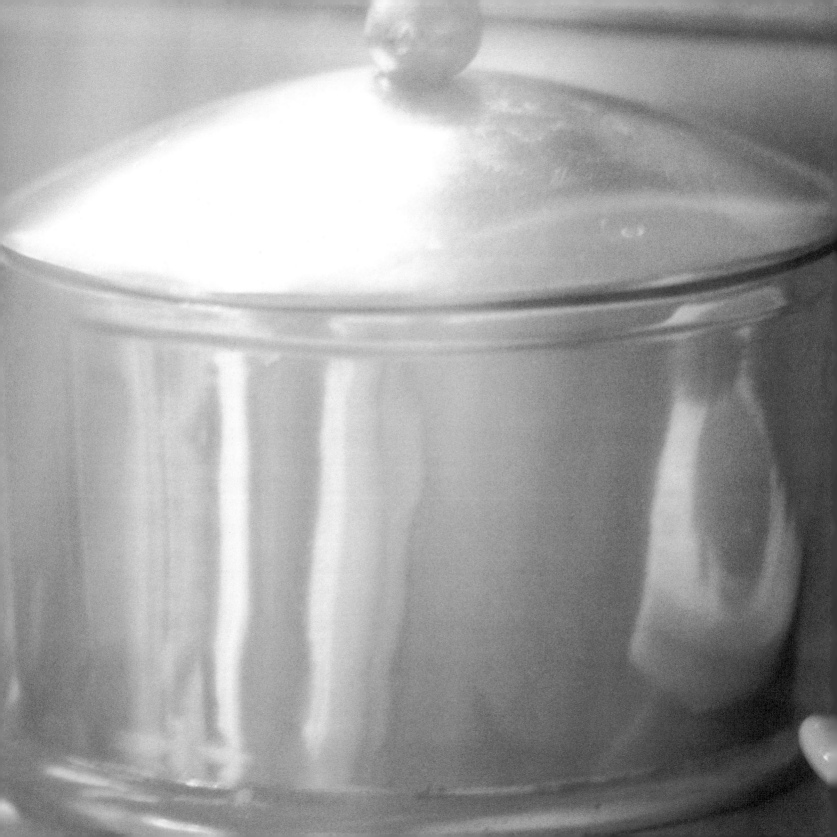

Birdbath   One comes across them on a gray, not-quite-spring evening, deep in the throws of it—dipping; splashing; and tossing back beakfuls of water over their feathery shoulders. Preening, gossiping, strutting, and generally bullying one another until the biggest or baddest ends up with the whole puddle to himself. Then suddenly, he can't bear the solitude and calls the others back. What a springboard for the spirit!

Moon Bath   She could not tell where the water stopped and her body began. The dog wanted in. The moon wanted in. It was the first gift he gave her—the lightly scented water, lapping, the silver rim of the moon in view. Nothing's like the moon but the moon, she thinks, as he washes her back. And she wonders what it might be like to take a bath there, in astral light, on a lunar sea … difficult to hang onto the soap, she suspects. It was then she realized the magnitude of his gift. And the world drifted off, lazily, the way a straw hat might float downriver.

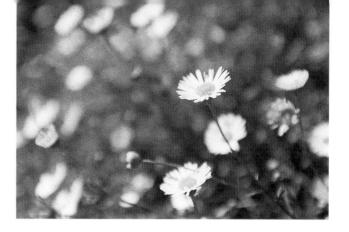

herbal hair rinse

Freshly brewed teas are terrific for rinsing freshly washed hair. It's a great way to apply scent without being too perfumy.

Brew two-cup batches of teas from either loose or bagged teas. This is a great way to experiment with your favorite brews. Here are some suggestions to get you started.

Chamomile: good for any color hair.

Lemon spice: great for blondes.

Peppermint: leaves scalp tingly.

Lavender: a crown of fragrance.

Green Tea: smokey, clean aroma.

flea tea

For all the dog lovers who enjoy the act of bathing human's best friend and keeping the fleas at bay.

A handful of fleabane (erigeron)

6–8 eucalyptus berries

A few sprigs of pennyroyal

A few sprigs of rosemary

Tie in cotton gauze and place in tub.

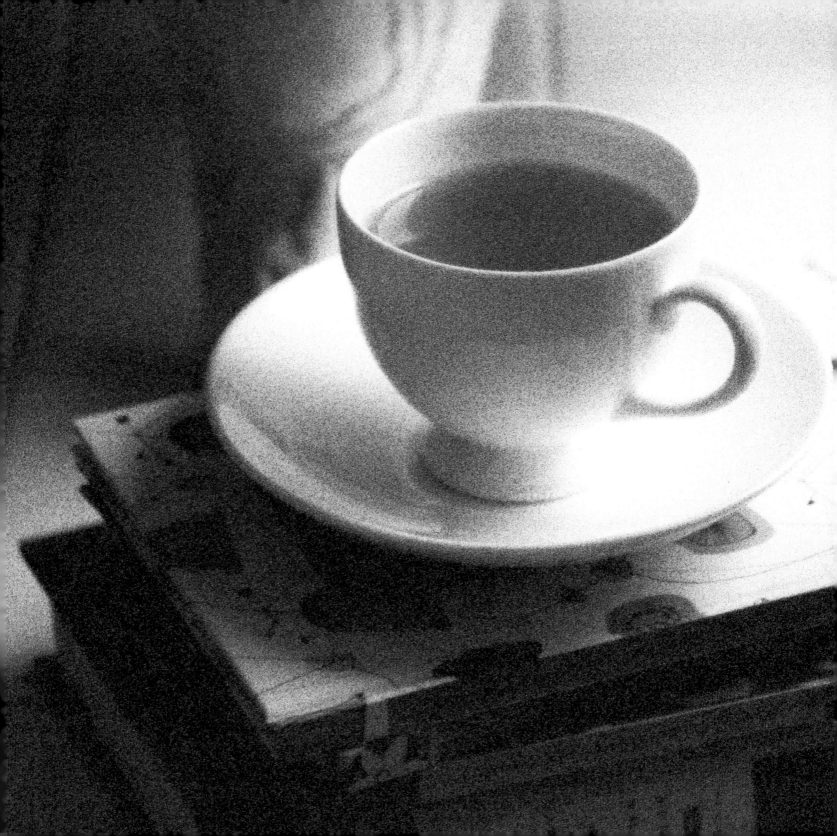

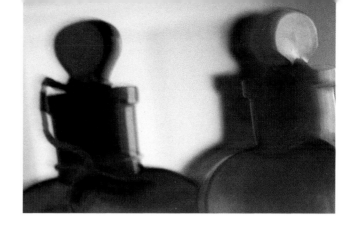

lemongrass and thyme tisane

Even though this tisane is a remedy for calming a cough and easing a hangover, it has a unique and elegant aroma. Soothing to sip and good for the body.

3½ cups of water

1 4-inch stalk fresh lemongrass

1 handful fresh thyme

Boil the water. Cut the lemongrass in half lengthwise and then in half again, so that you have long strips. Gently bruise the strips with a mallet or any hard object. This will release the fragrance. Place the lemongrass and thyme in a teapot with a strainer spout. Pour water over the herbs and allow to steep for 8 to 10 minutes. Serve warm, not hot; this will enable the fragrance to surface. Serves 2 to 3.

steamed cinnamon and lemon milk

Warm steamed milk will relax those frayed nerves. This is a drink your Mom gave you to make you feel special.

1½ cups low-fat milk

½ teaspoon fresh lemon zest

¼ teaspoon cinnamon

Place all ingredients in a milk steamer and steam until frothy. Pour into a warm mug or small bowl. Serves 1.

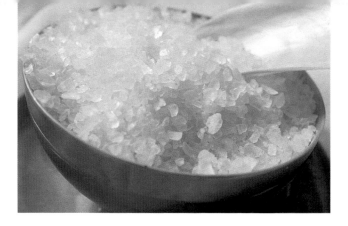

sea spray

A mineral-filled blend to soothe and relax muscles.

A handful of Epsom salt

A handful of seaweed or kelp (try a Japanese market for this)

5 or 6 ¼" slices of fresh ginger

baby bath

Baby baths are soothing and therapeutic for both baby and the fortunate person giving the bath. Since the baths are so portable this is a perfect opportunity to bathe baby on a deck or lawn, by an open window when a summer breeze is blowing, or even in the kitchen sink.

A handful of fresh chamomile blossoms

2 handfuls of calendula flowers

6 fresh rosebuds, crushed

1 spray of honeysuckle

Place ingredients in a large mesh ball or tied cotton gauze and let baby splash away. Dry off in warm, lavender-scented baby towels.

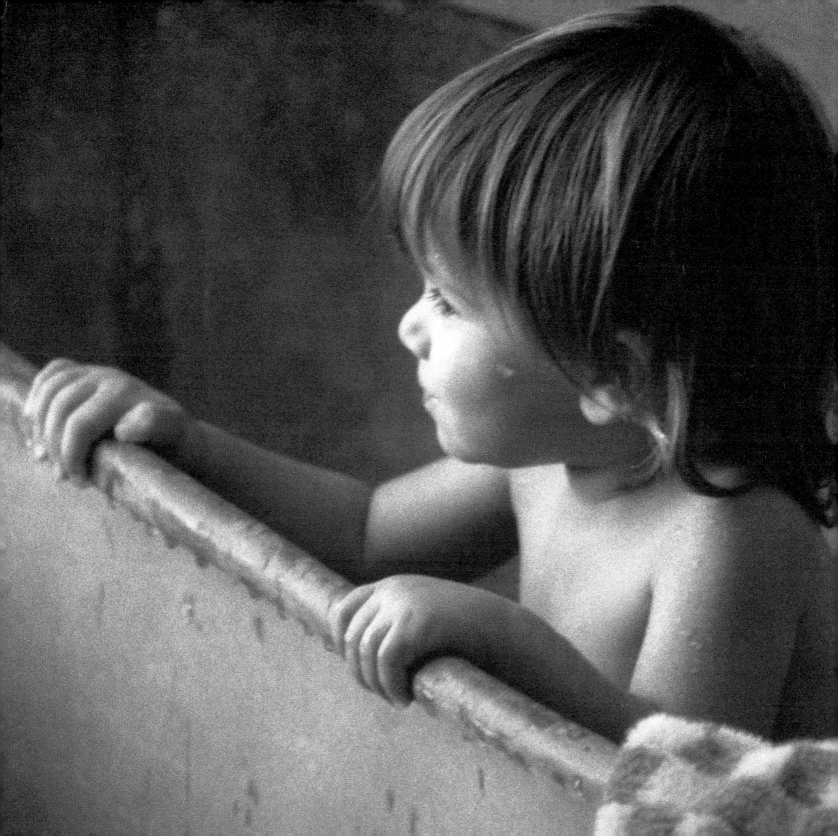

edible recipes

bath recipes